Take Control of Your Health

Take Control of Your Health

An Instruction Manual

Richard Helfrich

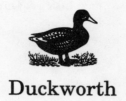

Duckworth

Fifth printing in 2007 by
Health Spectrum
149 Columbia Drive
Ranch Mirage, CA 92270

First published in 1996 by
Gerald Duckworth & Co. Ltd.
The Old Piano Factory
48 Hoxton Square, London N1 6PB

LIBRARY OF CONGRESS CATALOG CARD NUMBER: 2007940752

ISBN: 0-9661464-1-7

Other Books by Richard Helfrich

Immune Response

The 24 Hour Body

Young: Inside & Out

Printed In The United States Of America

Contents

x   *Contents*

Introduction

This book is dedicated to everyone who has the courage to take control of their body. We are all conditioned to rely on others, especially professionals who know more than we do. Each of us reaches a point in our life when we realize that there are no experts; it is usually at this point that we have to rely on our own instincts.

I would ask you to receive this book as an owner's manual for your body. I have laid out the precepts that will not only allow you to take control of your body, but more importantly allow you to begin understanding its functions and its incredible potential to be programmed or reprogrammed for health.

Even though each one of us is biochemically unique, we can by using this manual determine our individual blueprint. We are the sum total of two words: Chemical Reactions. I want to lift the veil of mystery by not bombarding you, the reader, with theory, but rather by providing protocols for a new life-style. By helping you understand how the body functions, its needs, its chemistry, I will enable you to anticipate your own unique requirements.

Let us together debunk conventional medicine that says we, the general public, are not capable of knowing what is good for us. Knowledge is power; and when confronted in the future regarding your health, you will not give your power away but be a co-participant in all questions regarding your health.

In 1981 I was diagnosed as having Cardio-Myopathy (CM), which by definition is a disease of the heart muscle. This condition had started with a heart murmur in my early teens, developing into an enlarged heart and a very irregular heartbeat in my twenties. I had gone into the hospital for a successful hernia operation, but before discharging me, the doctors decided that they wanted to do an EKG (electrocardiograph); this is when the fun began.

The appearance of a very irregular heartbeat worried my doctors and a cardiologist was called in. I began a battery of tests, the nuclear medicine ones being the most disturbing as they allow you to see your heart on the monitor in sections. I tried to tell the specialists that I had a low tolerance for this sort of thing: not only did I pass out, but I also went into convulsions. More than once I sent my shoe through the room, across the hall and into the next room.

The day of reckoning came. I had my audience with the cardiologist, who, by this time, had me on all sorts of medication, including nitroglycerine. After the predictable wait, he proceeded to tell me that the diagnosis was CM; I would be on medication from now on, and every few months would be brought in for a series of tests to monitor my condition. During his consultation he was constantly interrupted by the telephone. How lucky I was to be in my position, he told me, since the urgent calls he was taking were from people who were waiting for transplants. At least I would not be in that situation for a while; in the meantime they would simply monitor the atrophy of the heart muscle. The coup de grâce came when I asked the question, having no family history of this condition, what could have caused it. Probably an allergic reaction to alcohol, he opinioned, which left me finally speechless, since I barely drank alcohol.

I remember walking through the waiting room out of his office, looking at the people there, and thinking how they had all become victims; their lives, my life, were to be ruled by a cardiologist's dictates. How, and possibly how long, I would now live was now dependent on him.

This was the moment I chose to take responsibility for my body. I could not be at the mercy of a doctor's diagnosis of my condition and of his prescription for my health. I had to know what condition my body was in; and to do this I had to know my body better than anyone else. So with no knowledge, little understanding, but with determination and hope, I started a journey that changed my body and my life.

I ask you to take this journey,
to own your body.

1

Where do We Begin?

This book is not the be all and end all, but it will become the guide in the management of your health. The fact that you are reading this book in itself reveals an interest in hopefully a commitment to knowledge about your body. Many great books on this subject have been written already and these I will reference and recommend as additional resource material where appropriate. There are some areas I will touch upon, and others I will treat in-depth depending on the practical application of the knowledge. This book at all times is meant to be an owner's manual, so think of it as you would an owner's manual for your car. It will tell you how to turn the switches on in your body, but it will not explain all the intricacies involved in the engineering and make-up of the switch. Again that back up information, should you require it, is referenced where appropriate.

I want to begin with the first time I walked into a health food store, looked around, and thought, 'Oh My God! All these different supplements, how will I ever figure it out.' Well, that was fifteen years ago and I did figure it out.

What I am going to impart to you in this book is fifteen years of trial and error, of research, of listening and reading everything, and gleaning from all that what worked. As beneficiaries of this knowledge, I hope to speed your process to perfect health.

Most of the work I have done in the last few years has been with life-threatening illnesses. While I have personally found this work the most rewarding (and I will follow this book with a book specifically dedicated to treating life-threatening illnesses), the theme for this book developed when I found that people who were facing a terminal condition were much more willing to change their life-styles in order to heal themselves.

Most people with chronic or acute conditions are not motivated enough or else feel too overwhelmed by what's involved to make the commitment. But I also remember being in that position and wondering whether there was a book that could serve as a template for my own research? Unfortunately there was not, which required a lot of reading and researching into what was available, and then piecing the relevant information together. This created even more confusion, until I came to the conclusion that I needed to approach the body from a scientific perspective to find out what makes it tick. In doing so I found it much easier to cross-reference information from a body function perspective, extract that which was applicable, and discard the rest. There were a lot of startling discoveries, especially in how the body functions and what it needs daily in order to operate effectively and efficiently. This became more apparent once I started working with people, and came to appreciate their complete lack of understanding of their bodily functions.

So it is here that we begin.

2

Food

This vessel that we have been given to use during our lifetime, how incredible it is. Its ability to function on so many levels, spiritual, mental and physical. Today everyone seems to be willing to take responsibility for their spiritual and mental health – with countless support groups available and the growing awareness of the necessity to confront and understand old hurts and damage – as a prerequisite for healing. It is now physical health that we need to understand more and take responsibility for, so that when it is affected we know the action responsible. We need to debunk myths, conjecture and speculation, and to replace them with knowledge. We no longer need to operate without a manual; we now have access to the information necessary for reprogramming our bodies for health.

We need to understand that the body is a living, walking, biochemical laboratory with a computer system far superior to anything created by man, and that its long term functioning and the quality of that functioning is a product of the food it is fed.

When asked most people say: 'I eat healthy', 'I don't need supplements', and 'I get everything I need from the food I eat.' Sorry folks, wrong answer! The food we eat is so devitalized that we receive about 30% of the nutrients there were in the same food a generation ago due for example to acid rain, which blocks out absorption of selenium in foods that are supposed to contain this valuable anti-oxidant mineral. Often you will hear: 'My parents or grandparents lived until they were in their 80s or 90s'. But they were not raised on supermarket diets of preserved, processed food, and for the greatest part of their lives they primarily ate food that was not devitalized as it is today.

And what was the quality of their later years? If you have any doubt on this point please read *Diet for a New America*,[1] which gives a chilling account of most commercially grown food.

We can no longer rely on the food we eat to provide us with all the nutrients our body demands for its daily function.

People then say: 'But I'm taking supplements. I don't know if I feel any different.' Suffice it to say that the vast majority of people taking supplements get little or no benefit from them. Why? Wrong food combining and an etiquette that prevents digestion and absorption.

Chemistry is involved with every aspect of the body's function, especially when converting food to fuel. If there has been one constant over the years it has been the observation that besides genetic and environmental causes, diet and lack of digestion dictate most people's health. Even if we are eating a nutrient-rich balanced diet, and taking supplements, if digestion and assimilation are not taking place we are eating for the sake of eating. The first step to good health is proper food combining.

Food Combining

While a vast subject, with many books written on the subject, I want to establish a simple eating protocol that will form the foundation of your well-being.

First the food groups:

Vegetables

In their natural state or as close to it, where the living enzymes have not been killed through over heating, all leaf, root, and seed vegetables and sprouted seeds contain a resource of nutrients that includes vitamins, minerals and trace minerals. These provide not only nutrients but also neutralize toxic material in the body and flush out the large intestine, preventing impacted pockets of waste. It is important to remember that this group especially requires a lot of digestion for assimilation of nutrients and proper elimination to take place.

Proteins (Meats, Nuts, Seeds and Beans)

This food type forms the building blocks of our cellular make-up. Protein is somewhat of a misnomer: we don't eat protein, but foods that have the amino acids which allow our bodies to produce protein (discussed further in Chapter 6). These foods need a lot of digestion in order to release the amino acids and other nutrients, and should be eaten in moderation. Depending on your individual needs, some supplementation with digestive enzymes may be required.

Starches (Grains, Potatoes, Yams, Pasta and Rice)

This group we call complex carbohydrates, which the body breaks down through digestion, converts to simple sugars, and then stores as fuel. Less is more: the greater the quantity, the more the body has to work to accomplish this complicated task. Whole, unrefined grains are best, such as sprouts in breads, allowing the body an easier time identifying and processing.

Fruits (Acid and Sub-Acid)

These provide the best daily cleanse that you can give your body; but only until mid-day. After that time the body requires fuel from the other groups. Again, eat these in moderation and be careful with combinations. Be especially aware of orange, grapefruit and pineapple juices; because of their high acid content, in many people they may cause a negative reaction (moodiness, irritability, bloating, etc.).

When you buy your fruit and vegetables and are unsure if they have been sprayed or treated, soak them in a sink full of cold water for 10–15 minutes, adding a tablespoon full of non-chlorine bleach. This will neutralize all chemicals without contaminating the produce. Then rinse with cold water.

Simple Carbohydrates (Honey, Raisins, Dates, Figs, etc.)

These provide quick fuel for the body. No digestion is required, so they pass through the stomach very quickly, and are best eaten an hour before a meal. If you are working out, these are good energy foods. Moderation is the operative word, especially if you are addressing hypoglycemia or a diabetic condition.

In terms of combining, the following are the parameters you need to be aware of to address the next phase, digestion. Proteins mix best with vegetables. Starches also combine well with vegetables. Proteins and starches are poor combinations. Sweet fruits (bananas, dates, figs, etc.) mix well with sub-acid fruits (pears, plums, apples, grapes, etc.), but not with acid fruits (pineapple, oranges, grapefruits, lemons, etc.). Sub-acid and acid fruits mix but you need to limit the number of different types.

The easiest way to understand food combining is to look at food as enzymes, each food type representing a different type of enzyme. These enzymes become catalysts for different chemical reactions in the body, so it becomes very important to understand how every food affects our body. Because it is impossible to know how every single food affects us, we break them down into like/kind groups.

Let me give you some of my own recommendations for an average day:

Breakfast

Juice – nothing acid, in other words no orange, grapefruit or pineapple, instead try papaya, apple, pear etc.
Cereal – fat free if possible, without sugar
   – use apple sauce to sweeten
   – substitute milk with Rice Dream (made from rice) or soya milk.

Toast or muffin – again fat free and sugarless; toast cannot be burned
     at all, as the burned debris creates free radicals in the body.
     – use sugar-free jam, all fruit, and preferably non-acid.
Cleansing or detoxifying is a very important part of our body's daily
routine, and simple carbohydrates (fruit) only until mid-day allows this
process to take place.

Lunch

This is where you introduce your first amino based or protein foods of
the day.
     Salads – no iceberg lettuce (extremely hard to digest and of no
nutritional value).
     Grains or rice – Tofu, Tempeh or other soy products which can
replace meat.
     Vegetables – preferably root vegetables, lightly steamed, nothing
fried.

Dinner

Grains (pastas) or rice.
Salads.
Vegetables.
Meats (preferably meat substitutes).
     Between meals, but not before an hour has passed since your last
meal, try to drink at least 16 – 32 ounces (2 – 4 glasses) of water
(filtered) before your next meal. A critical requirement for flushing out
our second respiratory system, the lymphatic system, is to drink up to
64 ounces (8 glasses) of water each day – this does not include other
beverages. But timing is everything, and you should restrict your fluid
intake during meals to no more than eight ounces. This is explained in
Chapter 3.

Beware of these foods

     Tomatoes – have a unique acid all their own and do not mix well,
preferably to be eaten by themselves.
     Cooked spinach – while raw spinach is excellent, full of nutrients,
cooked spinach releases an enzyme that attacks the stomach lining.
     Artichokes – acts the same way as spinach, releasing an enzyme that
attacks the stomach lining.
     Mushrooms – try to avoid, because they contain a lot of yeast and a
high bacteria count.
     Melons – also have unique enzymes that do not mix well, definitely
eat by themselves.

Corn or corn flour products (especially chips) – very hard to digest. There is a reason the Europeans only fed corn to livestock – they have the stomach for it.

Peanuts – a definite 'stay away from'. Apart from being extremely hard to digest, they have a mould (Aspergillis flavis) that attacks the stomach lining. This mould, which is also found on corn products, produces a powerful carcinogen, aflatoxin, a known cancer causing agent.[2]

Again I also recommend reading *Diet for a New America*, an excellent expose of the poultry, beef, pork and dairy industries. If this information does not change your diet, then I doubt if anything will.

Having not come right out and said it yet, this seems to be an appropriate moment. We are talking about food combining, but what is the objective? Not only to control our consumption, but also to understand the effect of that consumption. So while I advocate a vegetarian or vegan life-style, I also believe in moderation and accept that not everyone can or will give up meat, dairy products or fish. But what I do want to impress you with is the effect of what we eat on the body.

Our digestive tract was not designed to deal with sustained quantities of (especially cooked) meat, poultry and fish. If a comparison was to be made, we as humans have a digestive make-up closer to primates (monkeys, apes) who are fruigivores. Carnivores such as the tiger (cat family) and wolf (dog family) are equipped differently from humans to deal with their raw flesh diets:

They have long, sharp teeth and jaws that only go up and down.
Their saliva is acid, necessary to digest flesh.
Their intestines are only three times the length of their trunk, for quick digestion and elimination.

Humans and primates on the other hand have:

Smooth teeth and a jaw that grinds sideways.
Alkaline saliva for digesting starches and carbohydrates.
A digestive tract that is twelve times the length of the trunk.

These basic characteristics and the precepts of food combining demonstrate that our evolution as carnivores was not by design.

Liquids

Water is our mainstay, as the body is composed of approximately 70% water. Vegetable or green drinks and fruit juices are also good sources of liquid. They are assimilated into the body very quickly, are full of living enzymes, and require little or no digestion. This is a great way to give the body a rest and fuel at the same time. However stay away from carbonated or pasteurized juices and liquids with chemical additives.

Water is the primary catalyst for the major body functions, especially elimination through the lymph system. Our lymph system is our second respiratory system and water is what flushes it out through muscle movement.

What kind of water?

Filtering water, either by a natural or man made process, removes most impurities. Tap water for the most part is chemically treated to remove impurities, but contains 50–60 chemicals, from sodium fluoride to chlorine, and must be avoided.

The safest and most body-friendly water is distilled water. Steam distilling not only removes impurities and bacteria but also draws inorganic minerals out of the body once it has been consumed. Be aware that bottled water can only be sold legally as 'Pure' or 'Spring' if derived from a natural source. These so called mineral waters contain inorganic elements such as sulphur, soda, magnesia, iron and lime. Over time, because of the body's inability to purge itself of these elements, mineral accumulation can cause harmful side effects such as arthritic conditions, organ stones or calcification, and damage to the circulatory system, especially the capillaries.

Always read the independent laboratory analysis of the organic and inorganic content of bottled water before purchase.

How much water?

At least 64 ounces (8 glasses) of just water per day excluding other beverages.

Wheat grass juice

I discovered this elixir in the late seventies and, since then, given the choice of just one complete food substance, I would choose wheat grass hands down. The chlorophyll found in wheat grass is almost perfectly matched to our blood, or, more specifically, our haemoglobin. The only difference is that the metallic atom of haemoglobin is iron while chlorophyll's metallic atom is magnesium.

Wheat grass juice is definitely the health connoisseur's drink of choice. Its list of benefits are practically endless, the primary are as follows:

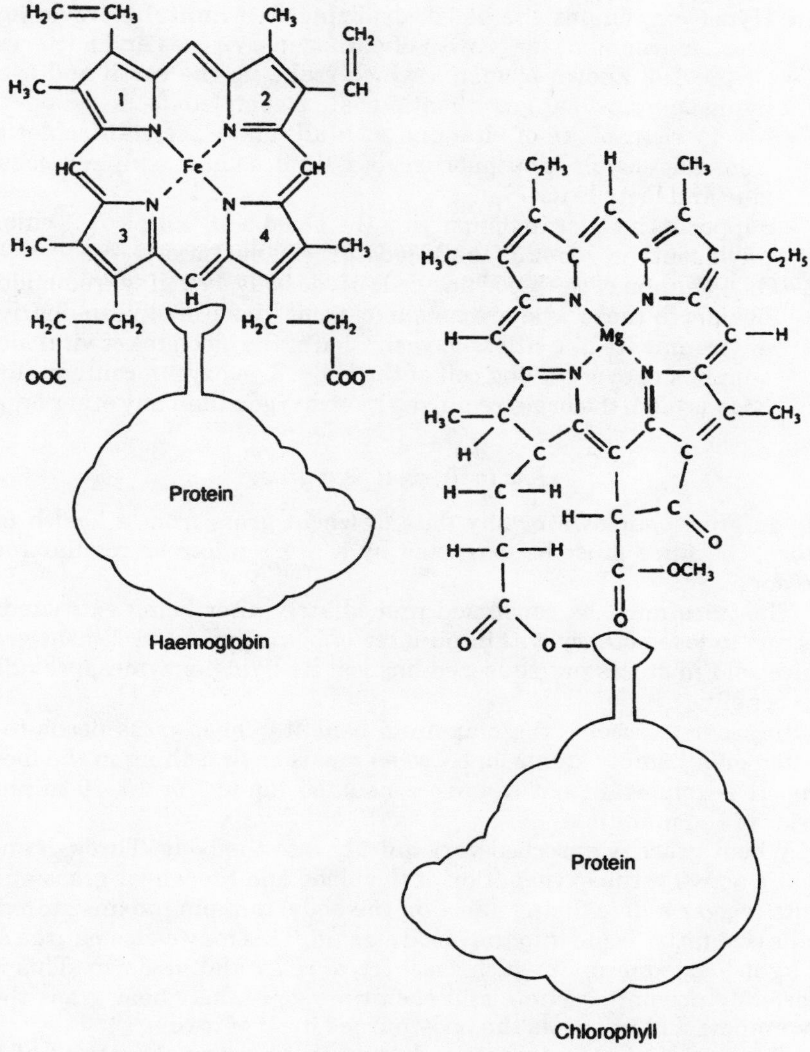

Figure 1. A comparison of chlorophyll and haemoglobin.

- Probably one of the best antibiotics, neutralizing micro-organisms.
- Hyper-oxygenates the blood, oxidizing free radicals, providing a poor environment for growth of pathogenic viruses and bacteria.
- Of the 103 known elements which make up the earth and every living thing, wheat grass contains all, a complete food.
- A very rich source of vitamins A, B(all) and C, calcium, chlorine, iron, magnesium, phosphorus, potassium, sodium, sulphur, cobalt, zinc and laetrile (B-17).
- Supports the liver in detoxifying the blood and, with a 70% chlorophyll content, rebuilds the blood at the same time.
- Oxygenation of the blood and cells of the body, bringing tremendous benefit to those who are anaemic, from living in oxygen-deprived environments like cities. Oxygenation of the blood takes vital blood supplies to every living cell of the body. The oxygen content of the body is 60%, the brain requiring more oxygen than any other organ.

How to drink wheat grass?

If you grow your own or buy flats of wheat grass from a health food store, the juice must be extracted by a grass juicer or regular meat grinder.

The juice must be consumed immediately after being extracted: it begins to lose potency within minutes of being extracted. Wheat grass juice sold in stores pre-squeezed has lost its living enzymes, providing no benefit.

In order to receive the maximum benefit, wheat grass needs to be taken on an empty stomach, between meals or first thing in the morning. It is important not to have consumed liquids for 15–30 minutes prior to consumption.

Wheat grass is absorbed very quickly into the body. Through enzymatic activity, the oxygenation of the blood and the wheat grass nutrients trigger a detoxifying effect on the body, dumping toxins stored in cells and fatty tissue into the blood stream. This may cause nausea and a light-headedness, in which case, try to relax and lie down. This is a perfectly normal reaction, and each time you take wheat grass these symptoms will lessen as the body purges itself of toxins.

There is probably no better detoxifier, so do not be afraid of the symptoms mentioned above; they should be no more severe than those we associate with hunger. This is the body's natural process of detoxification, activated when the stomach has been empty for up to eight hours. We typically think of nausea and light-headedness as hunger, when in fact it is a detoxification cycle, with the body trying to rid itself of toxins. Most people never give their bodies a chance to detoxify; the first sign of discomfort is interpreted as hunger, and the consequent consumption of food stops the detoxification process, and reverses it back to digestion.

Please keep in mind the most important point and argument for wheat grass: 'You Could Live on It'. I also recommend wheat grass as an implant, which I discuss in Chapter 4.

Rejuvalac – The Living Drink[3]

The pause that refreshes, that is rejuvalac. A fermented liquid made from wheat berries, it is probably one of the most user-friendly substances we can put in our bodies.

Enzymatic action is the precursor to all body functions. When the bulk of the food we eat is cooked, having no living enzymes, the body has to produce enzymes to process the food. In order to do this it takes enzymes from the immune system, leaving it under-equipped to fight assaults on the body by free radical damage and infection, and unable to properly heal itself.

Rejuvalac is a one-stop enzyme supply with pre-digested protein and Lactobacillus bacteria (friendly bacteria). As a pre-digested liquid it is effortlessly assimilated by the body. It is rich in eight B vitamins, vitamins E and K, proteins, carbohydrates, dextrin, phosphates, saccharines, Lactobacilli, Saccharomyces and Aspergillus oryzae. Amylases are derived from the Aspergillus oryzae and have the ability to break down the larger molecules of glucose, starch and glycogens during digestion. (Food research chemist Dr Harvey Lisle did this nutrient research on rejuvalac.[4])

Very effective in providing a friendly bacteria environment in the body, rejuvalac contains natural lactic acid and fermented enzymes which enhance metabolic action. By providing a bacteria friendly environment for Lactobacillus bifidus to grow, lactic acid is produced, which maintains the large intestine in a healthy environment where unfriendly bacteria and yeast infections like Candida cannot survive.

ENZYMES! ENZYMES! ENZYMES! – that's what it's all about. Enzymes are the fountain of youth and play a dramatic role in the three principals of life: assimilation, respiration and elimination. The protocol of eliminating waste from our bodies to the cellular level, providing the vast nutrient base that the body requires daily to fund the tens of thousands of chemical reactions, and oxygenating our blood so that it reaches every cell, constitutes the fountain of youth. When the body is not expending 100% of its immune system fighting free radical scavengers, and instead is repairing, healing and keeping cells alive longer, the aging process decelerates.

There are a number of ways to prepare rejuvalac. I use the following:

1. Using organic wheat berries (soft pastry wheat), rinse and then skim off the seeds that float to the surface.
2. Using spring or distilled water at a ratio of two cups water to one cup wheat berries, place in a mason or wide mouth glass jar.
3. You can use fresh cut blades of wheat grass on top of the water for filtering (optional) or a piece of muslin. After 48 hours, pour off rejuvalac. It will keep several days if refrigerated.
4. Pour two cups of water back into jar, allowing water to ferment only 24 hours. You can repeat this process once more for 24 hours before starting again with fresh ingredients.
5. Temperature is important, room temperature is best. If the environment is warmer, decrease fermenting time by six to eight hours.

Rejuvalac, unlike wheat grass, can be consumed with other solids and liquids, since it is a digestive aid. I also recommend adding other juices to give it flavour, but suggest that they be non-acid. Rejuvalac is an excellent alternative to water with a meal because instead of diluting digestive enzymes and hydrochloric acid it promotes digestion.

There are many other living food alternatives and elixirs that you can choose from, but rather than try to provide a list, I suggest that you refer to the books of Dr Ann Wigmore. Apart from her work with living food therapy, she also has many low cost techniques for growing and sprouting your own living food, along with countless recipes for living food dishes. While I have many personal favourites, I would ask you to enter this world of living food, experiment with the various recipes, and find your own preferences. Foods to look for which are rich in enzymes, pre-digested protein, and Lactobacillus bacteria (friendly) include:

- Green drink recipes.
- Fruit and vegetable juices.
- Nut milks.
- Fruit salads and soups.
- Soups (vegetable/bean).
- Sprouts.
- Nut and vegetable loafs.
- Essene breads.
- Sea vegetable salads.
- Fresh fruit desserts.

3

Digestion and Elimination

I am devoting a complete chapter to two of the key body functions, because they are very misunderstood subjects. The fact is that most people are starving to death; not from lack of food, but from devitalized cooked, processed food and an eating protocol that does not allow nutrients to be digested or absorbed.

Digestion

Even those with a proper diet, including supplements of vitamins and minerals, often do not realize the full benefit because of a poor digestion etiquette. Proper food combining is the key to the chemical and enzymatic reactions that need to take place in order for the body to be properly fed. This chapter explains how nutrients are assimilated by the body; and how to ensure that critical assimilation takes place.

Everything starts with the first bite; actually before that bite, because our saliva can start flowing at the anticipation of food. We have all heard the expression 'mouth watering'; saliva begins flowing and with it the enzyme ptyalin[5] (amylase), which begins the process of breaking down starches into simple sugars. This is also one of the reasons why chewing our food thoroughly is so important, not only to break it into smaller particles but also to mix saliva into it.

Once swallowed, the oesophagus produces a peristaltic wave that carries food into the stomach. The stomach is the point of collection where, through the body's incredible computer system, the food substance is identified. It is through this identification process that all sorts of chemical reactions take place.

Simple carbohydrates (fruits, etc.) require no digestion. Liquids also leave the stomach very quickly. But complex carbohydrates, proteins and fats will stay in the stomach for three to five hours. The stomach is lined with millions of tiny vilii (similar to coral), which are also found in the small intestine. Once food is identified a signal sent from the brain releases hydrochloric acid into the stomach. This is the only acid the body produces; the stomach lining is protected by an alkaline mucus coating to neutralize its effect, except on the contents of the stomach. This is a critical stage, because if the body does not produce enough hydrochloric acid (which most people do not) or if it is diluted through ingesting too much fluid with the meal, this initial breakdown of the food substance will not take place. To exacerbate the situation most people follow their meal with desert, by which time hydrochloric acid has already been introduced into the stomach. This combination of hydrochloric acid and simple carbohydrate sugar is particularly explosive. Not only have you ensured that very few if any nutrients will be realized from the meal, but also the food will stay in the system for twice the time involved in normal digestion; and because of putrefaction from food sitting in the system, gas forms, causing discomfort and auto-intoxication of the system. The stomach also produces the enzyme pepsin (which breaks down proteins and needs hydrochloric acid as a catalyst), renin, and a protein substance known as intrinsic factor, which serves as a neurotransmitter of B12 through the small intestine.

Enzymes are an important part of what takes place in the stomach, and enzymatic activity has the same requirements of hydrochloric acid. Eating foods that have living enzymes helps the stomach to accomplish this critical first stage of digestion.

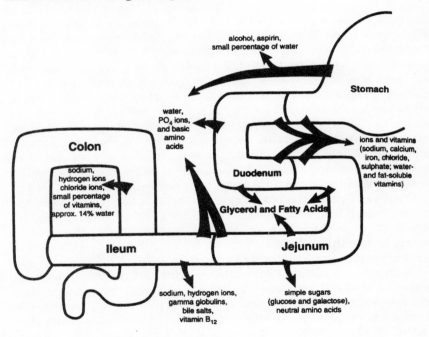

Figure 2. Absorption of nutrients from the digestive system.

As food leaves the stomach it enters the duodenum, a curved tube that is approximately the same length as the oesophagus. This is where food, that hopefully has achieved the first stage of digestion, is broken down further. Here the liver, pancreas and gall bladder all participate: the liver produces bile which is stored in the gall bladder and is released into the duodenum separating fats so that the pancreatic enzymes can break them down into a water soluble form that the body can assimilate. Bile also helps in the absorption of fat soluble vitamins A, D, E, F and K, and the assimilation of calcium, as well as converting beta-carotene into vitamin A.

The pancreatic enzymes, amylases, lipases and proteases neutralize the hydrochloric acid to produce the alkaline environment necessary for absorption, and further break down proteins and carbohydrates. The pancreas also secretes insulin into the bloodstream, regulating the burning of sugars in the body.

The next twenty feet of intestine is where digestion is completed, in the jejunum (approximately 10 feet) and ileum (10–12 feet). It is here that almost all absorption of nutrients takes place, and, if the environment is right – given the earlier stages provided the proper breakdown – that enzymes will have broken down the food molecules into a size that the billions of vilii or cells lining the small intestine will assimilate as nutrients.

Now we have amino acids from protein, sugar from complex carbohydrates, fatty acid, glycerol, vitamins, minerals and cholesterol all entering the bloodstream; and then heading for the liver, the main routing system through the hepatic portal system. The liver stores vitamins A, B12, D and iron for use as the body demands. It metabolizes fat in the synthesis of fatty acids from amino acids and sugars, and the production of lipoproteins, cholesterol and phospholipids. It also oxidizes fat for the body's energy, and produces fat from excess nutrients to store in the fatty tissues of the body.

The liver detoxifies the blood of everything, from the ammonia produced in the intestines during digestion, to all toxic substances, i.e. alcohol, chemicals (food additives, preservatives), drugs, metabolic waste, etc. It then passes these neutralized substances to the kidneys for elimination.

The regulating of blood sugar levels takes place in the liver through the conversion of thyroxine, a thyroid hormone, into its active constituent. By creating the GTF (glucose tolerance factor) from chromium and glutathione, blood sugar levels are balanced. Sugar is stored as glycogen and then converted back as the body's energy needs dictate.

Of the many functions the liver provides in sustaining life, the production of protein is at the top of the list. By assembling the amino acids from digested proteins, the liver acts as a combination lock; requiring the essential amino acids, that need to be consumed, to work in conjunction with the non-essential amino acids the body produces in order for the liver to produce proteins – the proteins which forms muscles, acts as neurotransmitters, identifies cells, and produces the immune system's antibodies and receptor cells. From the 29 known amino acids, including the essential, non-essential and those produced by chemical reactions in the body, the liver produces the complete proteins that form the 50,000 different proteins and 20,000 known enzymes. (Please refer to Chapter 6 for a complete description of this important subject.)

Elimination

Food now moves from the small intestine to the ileum and then into the colon (large intestine) or caecum. A valve, called the ileo-caecal valve, operates at this junction, preventing backup into the ileum. The material entering the colon is primarily indigestible material, mainly cellulose, which enters the colon in a liquid state. During the next 10 to 14 hours these substances will be dehydrated and stored in preparation for elimination.

I want to spend some time in explaining the importance of the colon to our overall well-being. There is no way to rank our internal organs in terms of importance, each plays such a unique role, but the colon probably has the greatest impact on all of the body's functions.

The body dumps toxins from the lungs, liver, and blood into the colon. But the colon can also be the origin of infection that infiltrates and permeates the body. Understanding the function of the colon may not be as dramatic as saving your life, but it may explain some of the chronic conditions you experience and allow you to begin a lower gastrointestinal tract maintenance that could dictate your quality of life for years to come.

Refer to the iridology chapter (Chapter 5) and try to locate your colon. You will find the caecum, ascending and traverse colon circumventing the right iris just inside the autonomic nerve wreath, and the tranverse, descending and sigmoid colon circumventing the left iris. Looking at the strategic positioning of the colon, as the core from which everything extends, you will understand how the colon's inter-relationship with all other parts of the body determines its overall well-being. Referencing your iris against the iridology chart, look for inclusions and or fissures in the fibres of varying colour from dark (degenerative) to white, which reveal toxic deposits and indicate the beginning of tissue irritation.

To understand the dynamics of the colon we need to look at its four-part structure. Almost five feet in length from the ileo-caecal valve to the rectum and making up 20% of the complete intestinal tract, it is much larger in size than the small intestine and sits in a more fixed position. Forming an arch shape, it begins in the lower right abdomen

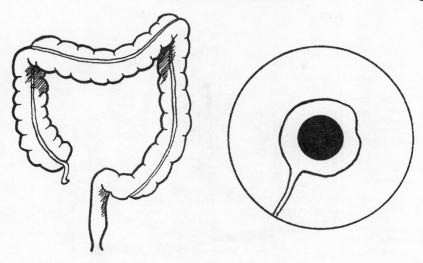

Figure 3. A healthy colon and its representation in the iris. Reprinted by permission of Dr Bernard Jensen.

ascending through the right lumbar region to just under the liver. There it bends to the left, passing across the abdomen (umbilical region) where it bends again, descending through the left lumbar region into the pelvis and down the posterior wall to the anus.

The colon wall has four layers: serous, muscular, areolar and mucous.[6] The serous coat is the membrane that attaches the colon to the perineum and the abdominal wall. The muscular coat is made up of longitudinal and circular fibres; the long muscle fibres forming the sacculi or pocketing. Within the muscular wall of the colon is the areolar coat, which connects muscular and mucous layers. The mucous membrane has a sub-surface of muscular layers with a layer of simple follicles similar to the villi of the small intestine. Interspersed throughout the colon, in the epithelium of simple follicles, are solitary glands, which consist of a dense tissue packed with lymph corpuscles, and a large capillary network providing blood supply to follicles.

There are two major grids of arteries which branch off to supply the colon and then divide into veins for the sub-mucous tissue and capillaries for mucous membrane. Known as the superior mesenteric artery and the inferior mesenteric artery, both emanate from the aorta and form the main routing system of blood to the intestinal tract.

The nerves that encompass the colon traverse the longitudinal axis and extend traversing within the circular tissue of the sacculated

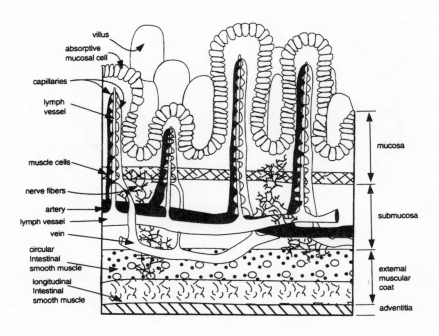

Figure 4. Cross-section through the intestinal wall.

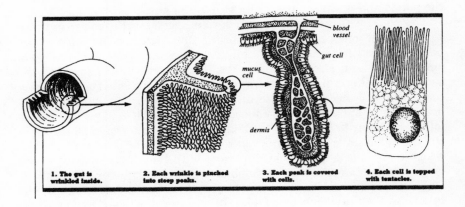

Figure 5. Cross-section of intestinal lining.

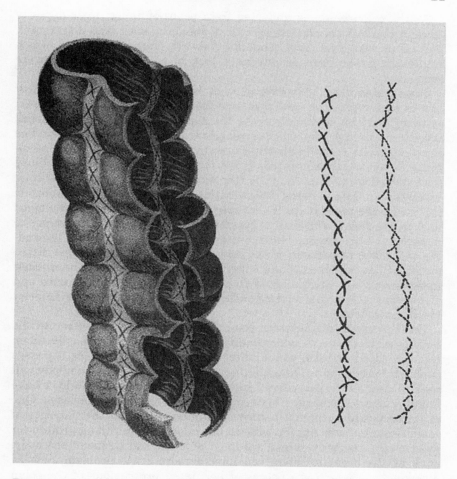

Figure 6. Left: Cross-section of healthy bowel, showing nerves and muscula-ture. Right: Drawing of colon nerve structure. Reprinted by permission of Dr Bernard Jensen

pockets. This nerve structure is probably one of the poorest of any organ in the body. Consequently the colon can develop spasticity, ballooning, diverticuli, etc. before we even notice. Gas problems can become so chronic that we accept it as normal, unaware of the damage to our colon.

Now that you have a general understanding of the digestive tract and in particular the colon, you can understand how we would almost be better off without the colon. This sounds quite radical, but given the average person's diet or life-style the colon becomes the breeding ground for all sorts of problems.

As the colon becomes impacted from years of abuse, toxic deposits form in the soft sacculated pockets of the colon wall (the diverticuli). The colon wall gradually loses its elasticity from distention, which results in tissue damage due to a lack of oxygen and other acute conditions.

How can so much go wrong in what is a five foot tube? The answer lies in understanding how that five foot tube actually functions. Its primary purpose is to dehydrate the material that leaves the small intestine, through the mucous membrane that lines the colon. The simple follicles discussed earlier are covered with a perforated membrane layer which allows the colon to release waste from the blood transported by the artery grids (the superior and interior mesenteric arteries). As fluid is being drawn out of the waste into the membrane this exchange takes place. There are two grids of veins that take blood back to the heart, and then to be filtered by the kidneys. The superior mesenteric vein returns blood to the small intestines, caecum, ascending and traverse portions of the colon and corresponds with the distribution of the branches of the superior mesenteric artery. The inferior mesenteric vein returns blood from the rectum, sigmoid flexure and descending colon, and corresponds with the branches of the Inferior Mesenteric Artery.

So the correlation between the colon and its systemic effect on the body is a direct one. A toxic condition in the colon can be easily taken into the blood stream, which, after doing tissue damage as it passes through major organs (heart, kidneys, liver, spleen, etc.), the body will seek to deposit. In the years I have been working in this field, I have found a direct correlation between the bowel and many diseases. One example would be breast cancer in women, which in the majority of cases observed was attributable to the colon. The dumping ground for most toxins the body cannot rid itself of is the soft tissue of the body, such as the breasts. When you have a more acute problem such as diverticulitis, which are polyps of herniated protrusions of the colon wall caused by impacted waste, the risk is even greater. Not only will the toxins be carried into the blood stream as the lining of the herniated tissue deteriorates, but the colon wall itself will also become diseased. Colon cancer is a major killer today, and it is indiscriminate. People who have the best medical help available to them die from it; Audrey Hepburn is one such casualty.

Other conditions brought on by poor diet include constipation, environmental influences, gas pressures (formed from putrefaction and fermentation of food in the system, pharmaceutical drugs, antibiotics, etc.) and the following:

Spastic Colon

This is brought on by nervous tension, creating a nervous stomach, and causing a stricture or spasm in the colon. More than ever before we hear of spastic colon diagnosis, which can be directly attributable to stress in our lives. The severity differs in each person and depends on the stage of degeneration (chronic or acute), but what it means is a strangulation of the colon, constricting the ability of waste to move freely through the colon.

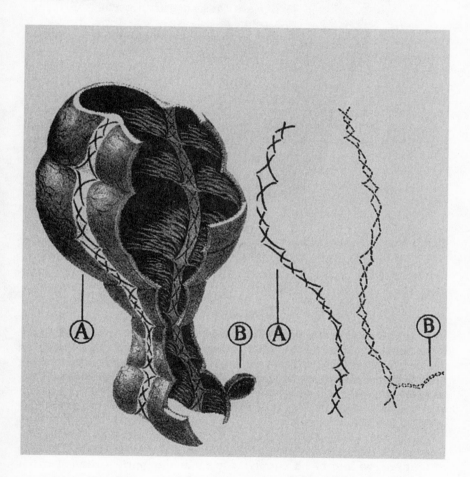

Figure 7. Left: Illustration of colon ballooning (A) and diverticulum (B). Right: Nerve structure. Reprinted by permission of Dr Bernard Jensen.

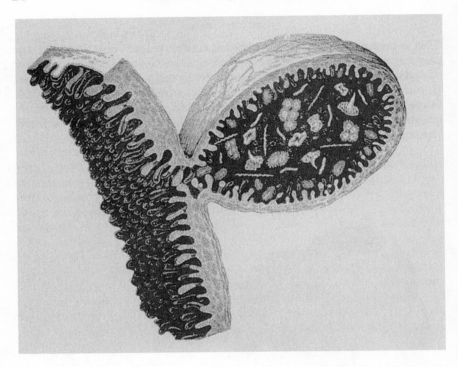

Figure 8. Enlargement of diverticulum, indicating toxins and bacteria impacted in colon wall. Reprinted by permission of Dr Bernard Jensen.

Diverticulitis

This is the more acute stage of a spastic colon. Portions of colon tissue have been damaged to the point where the colon wall has constricted making it extremely difficult for waste to flow through, and causing ballooning or distention of other portions of the colon before the stricture.

Colitis

This is a combination of both of the above in the acute stage. The lack of tone, nerve and blood supply to a particular part of the colon has inhibited the colon's ability to pass waste, resulting in a high toxic absorption rate.

Prolapse

This happens where a portion of the colon, usually the traverse segment, has collapsed. This is an acute condition brought on by lack of tone in the tissue, from constant irritation and lack of healthy tissue. It puts pressure on other organs, leading to further disorders, such as heart disease, lack of blood flow in the legs, etc.

Diverticulum of Polyps

This was discussed earlier as herniated pockets in the colon wall that trap waste. Because the waste is in a confined space with no flow through, as it breaks down over time it becomes very toxic. It damages the healthy tissue around it and ultimately leaks toxins into the blood stream which can be lethal when deposited in the organs and soft tissue of the body.

All of these conditions are reversible if the effort is made before the colon tissue is so damaged that the only option is a colostomy. If you are not having a bowel movement once a day at least, and preferably twice – one in the morning after rising and late afternoon or evening – you are in trouble. The longer waste sits in our system the more susceptible we are to auto-intoxication.

4

Colon Maintenance

Without understanding the digestive tract and its functions you will never be able to programme your body for health. I have found that the vast majority of diseases can be attributed in some way, shape or form to the digestive tract. Early in my journey back to health I heard about colonics or colonic irrigation. With much apprehension I investigated further; and it began to make perfect sense. The average American carries around 10–15 pounds of waste at any given time; due to our supermarket diets of processed foods up to 85% of the population is constipated to some degree and doesn't even know it; auto-intoxication is probably the first symptom of colon dysfunction and the early warning signal the body sends out. What is auto-intoxication? **The re-absorption of waste** (toxins) into the body: in other words a poisoning of the body. As discussed earlier, as waste sits in the large intestine it putrefies, and the longer it sits in the colon the greater the odds that the body will re-absorb toxins formed by this process. Aggravating this situation is the fact that the friendly and unfriendly bacteria levels are so out of alignment. The normal balance should be 80% friendly to 20% unfriendly; the reality is the opposite in the average person. As a result the friendly bacteria (acidophilic bacilli), which prevent or attack the effects of putrefaction and provide the acid environment that destroys bacteria, parasites, and Candida, becomes ineffective, and the unfriendly bacteria takes control. This exposes the body to all sorts of additional problems – such as parasites, which exist on most food that has not been washed properly or food that has been exposed to fertilizers made of manure. (Garlic is a very potent killer of parasites.) The E. coli bacteria epidemic at the *Jack in the Box* fast food chain is an example of this. Another major problem is Candida.

Candida albicans is a yeast like fungus that exists benignly in the mucous membrane of the large intestine. When the unfriendly bacteria environment is allowed to run rampant it activates and feeds the Candida, transforming it from a benign state to a destructive force in the body. Because Candida immediately upsets the body's chemical balance, it very quickly becomes immune suppressant, causing a worsening of conditions. What begins as a symptom quickly becomes a condition as the body chemically malfunctions to produce some of the following:

- Constipation, gas, irritable bowel.
- Food allergies.
- Psoriasis type skin conditions (rashes, nail infections).
- Arthritic conditions.
- Sinus drainage.
- Food cravings (especially sugar).
- White coating on tongue.
- Vaginal and urinary tract infections.
- Anaemia.
- Itching and perspiration.

The list could go on until it included almost every condition the body can experience; that is how pervasive Candida is. Each individual will suffer differently; because like any immune suppressant disease your body will attack itself where it is weakest. To eliminate Candida you need to mount an offensive: to remove the conditions that destroy the friendly bacteria and that starve the Candida of its fuel. This is like trying to put the genie back in the bottle; but it can be achieved. The protocol may include the following:

Drink rejuvalac (see Chapter 3).
Eliminate antibiotics, which destroy friendly bacteria in the body. (Ironically antibiotics are typically prescribed for the symptoms of Candida, while the Candida remains undiagnosed and the condition worsens.)
Eliminate birth control pills, which create hormonal disturbance, elevating blood sugar levels generally, and especially during menstruation.
Eliminate drugs used in cancer therapy, i.e. chemotherapy.

In addition starve Candida by eliminating the foods that fuel it, especially those with a high yeast or sugar producing content, and in particular the following:[7]

- No mushrooms (high yeast content).
- No fermented foods such as tofu, miso, alcohol.
- No vinegar, tomatoes, mayonnaise or mustard.
- No milk or cheese.
- No bread, cereal or pastas.
- No sugar or salt.
- No coffee or tea (even decaffeinated).
- No fried or canned foods.

• No fruits.

This may sound difficult, but the choice is yours: to live with the condition, or to change your life-style long enough to allow the body to take back control.

Daily Colon Maintenance

Fibre, fibre and more fibre, we need up to 60 grams a day. Fibre provides the lubrication the colon requires to function properly. Imagine a sponge that quadruples its size once wet, that's what fibre does once in the digestive tract without being absorbed.

Fibre falls into two categories: soluble and insoluble. The soluble fibre serves many functions, which include providing a conducive environment for friendly bacteria, slowing the absorption rate of sugars, lowering serum cholesterol levels, and binding to heavy metals dumped by the bloodstream into the colon.

Examples of soluble fibre foods would be apples, prunes, figs, raspberries, carrots, oat bran, kidney beans, lima beans or (supplemental) psyllium husks.

The insoluble fibre is the complement to the soluble, by increasing bulk in the waste, preventing impacted bowel pockets (diverticuli), reducing the length of time waste stays in the body and absorbing bile acid released during digestion. Examples of insoluble fibre are brown rice, quinoa, millet rice, whole wheat, raw spinach, brussel sprouts and flaxseed.

Fibre can make the difference between waste sitting in your system for up to three days or more, or 18–24 hours. Meats (red), chicken, fish, eggs and cheese have no fibre content, so the digestive tract has to work extremely hard to process them. Without fibre, these foods are going to stay in your system a long time.

One way to ensure an adequate daily supply of fibre is to supplement. There are a number of products marketed as intestinal cleansers, whose primary ingredient is usually psyllium. Not all are created equal and I have my own favourite, but whatever you take, make sure your water intake is sufficient to hydrate the fibre supplementation.

Colonic Irrigation

Also effective in the treatment of Candida are colonics. The primary benefit a colonic provides is the removal of impacted waste, gas, mucous and infectious toxic material from the large intestine.

The less waste the body has to deal with, the longer cells will stay alive and healthy. By removing the impacted waste from the colon we allow the tissue and the mucous membrane to breathe and to achieve the exchange of fluid and waste. With the removal of impacted waste, the colon is able to return to its normal shape, regaining elasticity and tone through oxygenation and increased blood flow. Like all conditions that develop in the body, developing into a chronic or acute stage, the cure or regeneration does not take place with one enema or colonic irrigation. An initial series is usually required to loosen and remove years of accumulation, then a maintenance programme of every month, or as dictated by your specific needs.

Colonics typically require going to a colonic irrigation technician. Holistic care clinics are also now offering the treatments. Through your local health food store or holistic care practitioner in your area or even your local Yellow Pages you should be able to locate someone offering colonic irrigation.

Do not be frightened or squeamish about the treatment, it is quite painless. The only discomfort you may experience will be from pressure during the filling process where the water is introduced into the colon. The procedure is very simple: a hose (sterile and non-reusable) with a 4"–6" attachment about half an inch in diameter is inserted into the rectum; the attachment has a single opening which connects to the hose outside the rectum; the hose brings water into the colon and removes water and waste. Most colonic apparatuses have a light box through which, as the flow is reversed, the waste may be observed, allowing the technician to identify various landmarks such as old faecal matter, mucous, parasites, undigested waste, etc. This serves an important function: enabling an experienced technician to identify and describe the problem areas and give a description of the colon's overall condition.

By repeatedly filling and emptying the colon as many as 6–12 times during a session, the colon is expanded and contracted, allowing old waste to be dislodged, pockets to be cleared and gas removed. After a treatment the recipient often feels energized and ethereal, as oxygen floods into the bloodstream.

If a colonic treatment is not available you can administer an enema with very little difficulty. Most drug stores sell hot water bottles with douche attachments that can be used for administering an enema.

Some simple tips when giving yourself an enema:

1. Make sure the water is cooler than room temperature; this causes the colon to contract, loosening old waste from the lining.
2. Have the water bag attached to a shower head. After inserting the water stem into the rectum, release the hose clip and kneel in a prone position with torso lower than the hips. Take deep breaths in this position.
3. Once water is inserted, remove the hose and lie on one side, rotating at intervals from side to back to side. Try to keep the

water in for as long as you can. You will feel the natural pressure to release, but with practice you can control this. Deep breathing, and massaging the colon to find the pressure points on the abdomen, helps.

4. After the enema, it is important to replace the friendly bacteria or, in most cases, introduce them into the colon. This can be accomplished by drinking rejuvalac or by taking liquid or powder form acidophilic bacteria (Lactobacillus bifidus).

When taking an enema always try to use distilled water, for the obvious reason that all impurities have been removed. Also you can add to the enema an ounce or two of chlorophyll (liquid) and/or flaxseed tea, to heal, nourish and reduce inflammation. Wheat grass introduced after the colon has been washed is also extremely healing. Once water from the enema has been eliminated, mix 4–6 ounces of fresh wheat grass juice (this requires being able to make your own at home) with 8–12 ounces of distilled water. Then using the enema bag introduce it into the colon, retaining the fluid for as long as possible. Your body will love you for this, and you will feel a bodily lightness as oxygen floods your bloodstream.

Please remember that most diseases can be attributed to the colon. It has been my experience, for example, that most breast cancer can be linked back to the colon. As toxins are carried into the bloodstream through auto-intoxication and from toxic deposits throughout the colon, the body looks to dispose of this material in the soft tissues of the body. In women the breasts are obvious targets. I am always amazed that this correlation is completely ignored and orthodox medicine's first reaction is to remove the infected tissue, and then irradiate to ensure success. Unfortunately, in most cases they have not addressed the problem but only temporarily eliminated the symptom. In time the problem resurfaces, and then it is usually fatal.

This is one example, but the correlation between the colon and disease could be made with almost every illness, even viral infections. We all have cancer every day; but what prevents the cancer cells from clustering, what keeps viruses dormant in our bloodstream, is a strong immune system. We do not have to wait for miracle cures from science. If we wait for vaccinations against HIV, herpes, hepatitis, or even the common cold (which is probably the most virulent of all these viruses) we abrogate the responsibility for our own health. Colonics are a step in the direction of taking that responsibility. It is the one procedure that done on a regular basis (depending on the individual condition) will, if not save your life, determine its quality.

5

Iridology

Early in 1982 at a Whole Life Expo in Long Beach, California, I came into contact with iridology. Dr Bernard Jensen, who was a speaker at the Expo,[8] had a booth, where a technician would photograph each eye, and two weeks later the analysis would arrive in the mail.

This chance encounter opened a diagnostic door that I have used ever since, not only on myself but also as one of the most reliable and direct ways of looking into the body. I urge you to become familiar with this science. It will change both the way you understand your body and the condition it is in, and how you look at other people. The cliché 'beauty is only skin deep' is truly represented by the iris, the window into the body.

When I look at the photograph of my iris as it was in 1982, its colour is mixed, full of nerve rings and it displays anaemia, lymph congestion, acidity throughout the body, mucus bowel pockets, and many more deficiencies. Compared with my iris today, with all these conditions eliminated and my eye colour brilliant green, it is as if the picture of the iris taken in 1982 belonged to someone else.

Iridology was discovered or first documented in the early 19th century in Europe. In this century Dr Bernard Jensen pioneered the science of iridology in the USA and developed the charts used today. These charts provide the important schematic that map out the entire internal body and all its functions in the iris.

How does iridology work?

Using the chart we see that each eye represents a different side of the body. The left iris, the left side of the body, the right iris, the right side of the body. The head is at the top of the iris with corresponding structural parts and organs in their proper order down to the feet located at the bottom of the iris. Symmetrical and paired organs like the kidneys are found in both eyes.

Imagine being able to access through a computer terminal display screen a picture of every aspect of your internal make-up – this is what iridology allows us to do. Every nerve in the body and the part of the body, to which it corresponds, is connected in the iris and bound by the autonomic wreath or nervous system.

If we further break the iris down into seven concentric circles, starting from the pupil and working out, we see the following:[9]

Figure 9

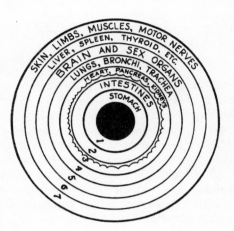

1. Stomach.
2. Intestines.
3. Major organs.
4. Interior of organs.
5. Exterior of organs.
6. Lymphatic and
   circulatory systems.
7. Skin.
Reprinted by permission of
Dr Bernard Jensen.

The whole digestive tract is the only part of the body represented within the area we call the autonomic nerve wreath. This is vital in understanding the major role the digestive tract plays in our overall well-being. Since the autonomic nerve wreath is the core or connecting point of all the nervous system, we see how the digestive and intestinal tract influence almost every aspect of the body. It is this connection that the irises have with the brain, the sympathetic nervous system and the circulatory system that provides us with this diagnostic printout of the body.

It is interesting to note that the iris colour or pigment is made up of nerve endings and is constantly replaced as the eye colour is maintained. For this reason researchers believe that the nervous response to stress, inflammation, toxic waste, drugs, injury, etc., causes alterations in the normal pigment or iris fibre structure.

The Diagnostic Iris[10]

When you look at the iris, imagine it as the sun with its central core and rays projecting outwards. The rays become fibres and in a perfect eye we see no flaws but only a fine even density. We call this the iris weave, reflecting the inherent constitutional strength and recuperative ability of the body.

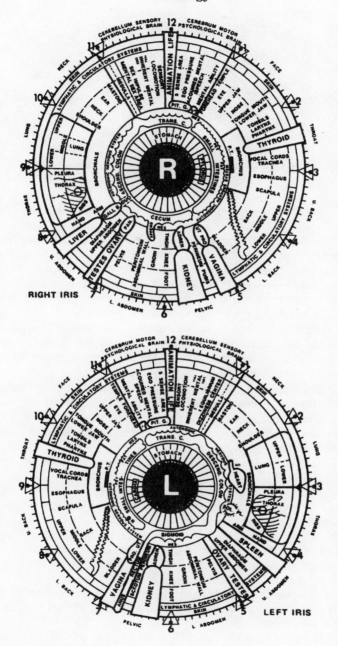

Figure 10. This chart represents a map of each iris, indicating organ and tissue location. Reprinted by permission of Bernard Jensen.

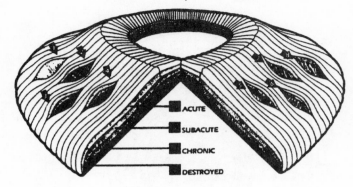

Figure 11. Side view of iris. Reprinted by permission of Dr Bernard Jensen.

If we look closer or at a side view of the eye we notice that the fibres seem to come out from the pupil joining the other part of the fibre coming in from the perimeter of the iris in a raised relief at the autonomic nerve wreath. It is this raised topography of the iris where we see the depth to the fibres. The top of the fibre will be white and get progressively darker as we approach the pigment layer.

Acute conditions, such as inflammation, congestion and injury will appear in the iris as a line (straight or distorted), flakes, webbing or clouds. Most of these indicate symptoms of recent changes in the body and if caught in time can be quickly reversed.

Darker inclusions represent more chronic conditions that have developed over time as a result of environmental effects on the body (i.e. pollution, stress, etc.) or genetic or inherent weaknesses in the body. The latter are much more difficult to address and require a concerted effort over a sustained period to reverse.

The typical chronic conditions show up in the iris in the following ways:

- A tear or separation in the surface fibres of the iris, exposing the underlying, darker layers of iris tissue.
- Webbing – where the iris fibres diverge in smaller large arcs, exposing the darker layer of the underlying iris tissue.
- Lymphatic rosary – a string of white spots in the concentric pattern in the lymphatic and circulatory zone.
- Radii solaris – isolated areas of small or large spokes, emanating from the intestinal tract, indicating routes of toxic build up and nerve weakness.
- Nerve rings – circular rings that dissect the iris fibres in a broken fashion almost like grooves on a record disc, indicating nerve damage and stress.

- Scurf ring – a dark circle that may affect one area of the perimeter of the iris or form a complete circle and vary in width. Indicates poor skin tone and eliminative vitality of skin. This is tied directly to lymphatic and circulatory function.
- Sodium ring – an opaque white ring clouding a portion of the perimeter of the iris, which indicates sodium and/or other inorganic minerals, or cholesterol that causes tissue to ossify (harden).
- Anaemia – a fuzzy or hazy rim usually at the top of the iris. Because the brain demands the most blood, a lack of circulation or quantity of blood supply shows up here first.

Healing signs are manifest in the form of white lines (calcium lutein) which, as healing takes place, form a grid over the dark fissure openings, knitting them back together with healthy tissue.

I have used iridology in my healing work and find it to be the most direct window into the whole body. I have never seen two people with the same iris, and, more the rule than the exception, have found very few examples of perfect health. There are a lot of people, however, who have been blessed with great genetics, or what we call a great constitution. They have the underlying star burst with a strong degree of density, which indicates excellent recuperative power and regeneration.

This sometimes works against individuals with a better constitution over people with a low density or weaker constitution. The person who has the stronger constitution will sometimes let a condition become acute, as opposed to someone who will become debilitated by the same condition in its chronic stage, when it is easier to reverse.

While not being able to identify a specific disease in its micro-cellular or biochemical distinction, iridology provides the road map for the diagnostician. This road map allows us to see where the weaknesses are and identify the inflammation on an energetic tissue level. We may not be able to tell when a heart attack may occur or the specific cancer that may manifest; but we will see the indicators that provide an early warning system.

I hope this brief overview will cause you to delve further into this amazing science. I urge you to pick up any of the books Dr Bernard Jensen has written on this subject, his most comprehensive being *The Science and Practice of Iridology* (see illustration). I recommend also Theodore Kriege's *Fundamental Basis of Iris Diagnosis*.[10]

Get a worksheet with the iris drawn, or draw one. Using the chart map out your own eye, starting with the landmarks you have become familiar with in this chapter. Then work backwards identifying your various iris components and see how they match up with (systemic) conditions you are already aware of. You will be amazed and, more

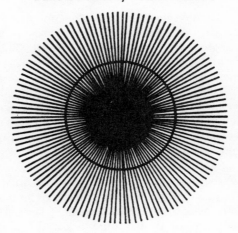

Figure 12. A worksheet. Reprinted by permission of Dr Bernard Jensen.

importantly, will be able to address specific concerns, rather than feel overwhelmed by all the symptoms.

A number of years ago the auto companies came out with a computerized system into which mechanics could plug your car to discover where the problems were.

Think of iridology in this way: your own diagnostic device.

6

Amino Acids

How do we rebuild the body?

If every cell in our body is replaced every seven years, other than our teeth, why do we age? What triggers the aging process? If the body has been completely replicated during a seven year cycle, why do we not replace atrophied tissue and organs with healthy cells? The answers to these questions lie with amino acids.*

Amino acids form protein in all living things; and human protein is the nucleus of all cell structure. It is protein that comprises, next to water, the largest part of the body's weight and substance. This includes our bones, muscles, tendons, internal organs, nails, hair, glandular functions, enzymes etc. Almost every conceivable structure and function of the body requires protein derived from amino acids to produce the 50,000 different proteins and 20,000 enzymes the body requires daily.

If you refer back to Chapter 3 on digestion you will recall that the liver produces the body's protein. Of the 29 known amino acids, eight are called essential and need to be consumed daily. Think of the liver as a combination lock that does not open to produce protein until all the amino acids are present and accounted for. Only then will the liver start producing the protein necessary for all the body's functions.

Remember that the body replicates itself every seven years and you will realize we are the result of chemical reactions. Amino acids allow tens of thousands of these reactions to take place daily, funding growth and repair. It is amino acids that allow the following:

The bone marrow to make 2.5 million red blood cells every second.
The lining of the gastrointestinal tract and blood platelets to be replaced every four days.

---

* For more information on amino acids see: Rose S., *The Chemistry of Life* (Pelican, London, 1985); Quastel, J. 'The Role of Amino Acids in the Brain', *Essays in Medical Biochemistry*, Vol 4, Great Britain, 1979, 1.48; Bodanis, David, *The Body Book* (Little, Brown & Co., 1984); Balch, Jr., James and Balch, Phyliss, A., *Prescription for Nutritional Healing* (Avery Publishing Group, Inc., 1990); Shabert, Judy and Ehrlich, Nancy, *The Ultimate Nutrient, Glutamine* (Avery Publishing Group, New York, 1994).

White blood cells to be replaced every 10 days.
New skin to be replaced every 24 days.

Without ingesting the essential amino acids daily, body functions begin to break down rapidly. (This traces back to what triggers the aging process.) Amino acids act as both precursors and neurotransmitters allowing the brain to both send and receive messages in up to fifty different chemical languages.[11] A sustained deficiency will not only preempt these transmissions, but short circuit the complete nervous system, wreaking havoc on the body's function.

The fact that some of us are born with genetic weaknesses or deficiencies also plays havoc with our overall well-being. Because of an inability to produce or absorb certain amino acids, we need to establish our individual requirements before we reach an acute state of health from years of producing incomplete chemical reactions. Think of the body as an assembly line that produces widgets: if you left out a screw last month, a nut this month, next month the widget would still be coming off the line but would fall apart the minute you tried to use it.

Amino acids are strategic to the body's functions as precursors, neurotransmitters and peptides, which form the chemical languages. When the brain communicates with organs or muscles, amino acids are the neurotransmitters. As precursors amino acids manufacture the chemicals necessary for the body to function; as do peptides, linking amino acids to produce hormonal and blood/brain chemical complexes.

In understanding amino acids, we can begin to unlock the body's chemistry. By utilizing amino acids we can correct deficiencies, reverse cellular or chemical based disease, and atrophy.

Do not be frightened: this is complex, but we are not aiming for a Master's degree in biochemistry. What I will recommend is that you look at your diet. It is not so much the protein based foods you are eating but how much available protein your body is utilizing from that food. The digestive tract has to work very hard to obtain amino acids, which takes us back to digestion and the correct conditions for nutrients to be absorbed.

There is an easier way. Instead of worrying if your body has extracted all the necessary amino acids from your diet, free-form amino acids in the form of supplements (preferably in powder capsules), taken correctly, enter the bloodstream almost immediately with very little effort on the part of the body. Without over-involving ourselves in clinical descriptions, the best over the counter amino acids are the L (left) form, which delineates the rotation of the molecules of the amino acid, and D (right) form amino acids which the body has to convert to L form to be used (other than methionine and phenylalanine in which the DL combination is optimum).

Multi-amino acid formulas versus individual amino acid supplementation

This is an individual choice. I have been taking a multi-amino acid formula for the last eight years. There is a school of thought which believes that multi formulas are ineffective other than for individuals with generalized deficiencies. Because of our individual biochemical uniqueness and the fact that our body requires the essential amino acids daily, I depend on a free-form formula to supply the essential and non-essential amino acids which allow the liver to produce protein on demand. Even this is no easy task, for the free-form (those that have been broken down into a form the body can assimilate) require neuro-transmitters and precursors to assimilate them into the blood stream. Once in the bloodstream they become part of the metabolic pathways, that your body determines based on its particular needs. Enzymes are metabolized to link different amino acids and hormones, but it is our DNA and RNA that actually direct this process of repair and rebuilding.

DNA (deoxyribonucleic acid) holds the blueprint for the entire body in its strands. DNA contains the information of body structure, RNA (ribonucleic acid) contains the metabolic index. If your body needs muscle fibre, RNA discovers the part of the DNA master plan that contains the information needed for the relevant piece of protein synthesis. The RNA then attaches itself to the section of DNA. The RNA assumes the shape of this part of the DNA, becoming an exact copy. This copy is known as a ribosome. Detaching itself from the DNA, it acts as a pattern for protein synthesis, attracting and binding the amino acids in the correct number and sequence according to the code it has copied.

I use the following formula, preferably first thing in the morning on an empty stomach.

Free-form amino acids
B-complex or individual B-6 (pyridoxine)
Vitamin C
Simple carbohydrate (juice – preferably non-acid, papaya, grape, apple, etc.)

B-6 is a co-factor which triggers the enzymes called transaminases to metabolize amino acids. I prefer a B-complex since B-2 (riboflavin) and B-3 (Niacin) are also required for metabolism.

Vitamin C also acts as a catalyst for metabolism. I take 500 mg of an ester C. As a vegan, I have found that this combination has literally changed my well-being. Prior to taking amino acids, I found it very hard to retain weight. I used to weigh about 148 lbs at 6' 1" which was rather light. I now weigh 180 lbs with little body fat and toned muscle. This

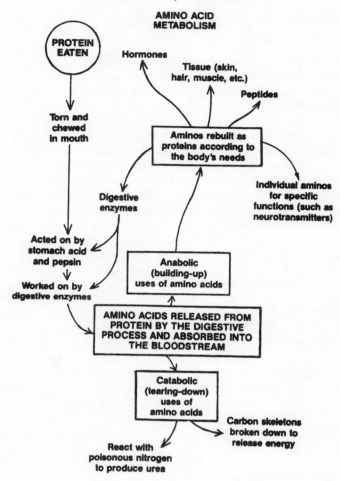

Figure 13. Amino acid metabolism.

formula has helped me build muscle tissue, not feed on it, as well as covering the maintenance of all the other body functions.

Depending on your individual needs, amino acid supplementation can be effective in fine tuning or addressing specific problems, such as anti-aging, heart disease, arthritis, stress, allergies, memory loss, depression, addictions, hair growth, and most other maladies you can think of. This is because amino acids are the building blocks of the body, affecting such fundamental biochemical structures as hormones, enzymes, the immune system, etc., and are the largest constituent of our cells.

If you think of the body as a living laboratory, amino acids are the fundamentals of the body's biochemical functioning. They are the greatest contributors to our well-being, and their patterns and deficiencies play a significant role in disease. And herein lies the secret: as we understand the body's chemistry, so we begin to learn how we can identify deficiencies by their landmarks and thus avert our individual biochemical malfunction.

So how do we begin this biochemical odyssey? Start by looking at the principles discussed in this book. How many of them apply to your present life-style? Then make a list of your general well-being, including all the conditions you would like to change, such as allergies, acne, hair loss, dry skin, warts, Candida, periodontal disease, migraines, stress, weight – the list of possibilities is endless. But your list is unique; and once you have identified all the problem areas that are taxing your immune system and overall well-being, you can, using amino acid therapy as one of the tools, begin to reprogramme yourself for health.

At this point I would like to mention that while working with people who have life threatening illnesses, I have never been able to address the illness without first addressing the chronic or acute conditions that have debilitated their immune systems in the first place. In other words there is no point rebuilding a car's engine unless you first repair the components that contributed to its breakdown. This section on individual amino acids will serve as a guide to rebuilding your own engine. Once you have charted your body's profile you can apply those amino acid therapies which address your specific needs. Please remember that research on amino acid therapies is extensive, and I encourage you to refer to other sources for further information.

Amino Acids = Amino (Ammonia) + Acid (Vinegar)

Ammonia or amines are the messengers, the neurotransmitters that provide the sparks for body function.[12] Acids are the fuel of body function and the detoxifier. Some amino acids are indispensable components of our diet.

The eight essential amino acids are:

1. L-lysine
2. L-leucine
3. L-isoleucine
4. L-methionine
5. L-phenylalanine
6. L-threonine
7. L-tryptophan
8. L-valine

L-phenylalanine

An essential amino acid found in bran proteins and blood plasma. Important constituent of many brain neurotransmitters, peptides, and proteins which form the brain's language for communication with the body.

Elevates our epinephrine levels, effective in treating depression – a precursor of adrenaline.

Blocks enzymes in the nervous system which break down hormones (endorphins, enkephalins) that elevate moods, acts as analgesics for pain associated with osteoarthritis, arthritis (rheumatoid), joint pain, menstrual cramps and headaches.

Used to increase alertness and stamina during athletics.

Certain cancers and melanomas have been considered to feed on phenylalanine, necessitating its exclusion from the diet i.e. no dairy products, or meat of any kind.

The best natural source from food: wheat germ, granola, oat flakes.

L-tyrosine

Can be manufactured by the body. Very important to brain nutrition, precursor to the neurotransmitters dopamine, norepinephrine and epinephrine. A pain reliever in the brain.

Precursor for production of the skin pigment melanin.

Ingredients of protein amino sugars and lipids which fuel body functions. Tyrosine helps the body cope physiologically with stress and building the body's natural store of adrenaline. Stress exhaustion needs tyrosine which converts to dopamine, norepinephrine (adrenaline) and tryptamine, all of which are the weapons the body mobilizes to deal with physiological and psychological stress. (I take 500 mg of tyrosine each morning with my daily ritual of amino acids, B-complex, vitamin C, etc., providing a great feeling of calm throughout the day. Even when dealing with stressful situations, there is a feeling of physical and mental detachment.)

It can be effective in controlling appetite and stimulating sex drives and is an effective anti-depressant.

Best natural sources from food: wheat germ, granola, rolled oats.

L-tryptophan

Removed from the market by the United States Food and Drug Administration (FDA) after a claim that it caused deaths due to hepatic coma (where the liver loses control of metabolic function). Interestingly it is now prescribed and administered in hospitals and doctors' offices.

Precursor of serotonin, a brain neurotransmitter, platelet clotting factor and neurohormone found in organs.

Effective in treating insomnia, reducing the time needed to fall asleep. Deep sleep disorders may be improved through doses clinically controlled.

Anti-depressant, also effective in treating manic and aggressive behaviour. It stabilizes blood sugar, reducing appetite for carbohydrates. Stimulates growth hormone and prolactin. In Parkinson's disease it inhibits tremors.

Can improve condition of kidney damage brought on by hypertension or uraemia.

Best natural source: wheat germ – 400 mg in one cup.

L-cysteine and L-glutathione

These are sulphur-based, non-essential amino acids. In Ancient Rome, injured soldiers were sent to sulphur springs or spas to heal their wounds. (There is one north of Rome, Saturnia, which was established BC and still operates today.)

Sulphur is antibacterial, and cysteine, which is a sulphur compound, acts as an anti-oxidant/antibacterial in the body, addressing auto-immune disorders such as rheumatoid arthritis and conditions from baldness to cancer.

Cysteine is used as fuel through a complex conversion into glucose or to be stored as starch. Cysteine also acts as a co-factor in the body's synthesis of fatty acids by the body cells for energy.

Cysteine determines how much glutathione, a powerful anti-oxidant and detoxifier, is produced by the body.

Findings have indicated that daily supplementation of cysteine increases hair shaft diameter and hair growth density. Also there is evidence that high sulphur proteins like cysteine are absent in people experiencing hair loss.

Cysteine is helpful in protecting lung tissue from the damage of cigarette smoke, especially the alveoli, the tiny sacs that make up the surface of lung tissue. Asthmatic and bronchial conditions, and their effect on mucous in the lungs and bronchial tubes are also aided by cysteine.

Glutathione plays a number of primary roles in protecting the body. It helps the liver to detoxify poisonous chemicals, provides several critical aspects of immune system function, and helps protect the integrity of red blood cells. It is also a neurotransmitter.

Glutathione can be especially effective for those exposed daily to slow rush hour traffic or polluted urban air (I live in Los Angeles where breathing the air has been equated with smoking a pack or more of cigarettes per day).

Remember that cysteine works synergistically in the body with vitamin C and other anti-oxidants, protecting cell membranes against oxidation of lipids, and in neutralizing pesticides, herbicides, hydrocarbons and drugs. It also acts as a bactericide, and as part of the glutathione molecule is an essential component of the immune system.

Best natural source: wheat germ, granola.

L-lysine

Found in large quantities in muscle tissues, lysine is a precursor to many of the body's chemical reactions. From forming collagen, the body's connective tissue, to helping the metabolism of protein, lysine plays many roles.

Clinically lysine has been used in recent years as an effective treatment for Herpes virus infections. This includes all variations, oral and genital, both Herpes simplex I and II. Most treatments include zinc, vitamin C, bioflavanoids and lysine working synergistically.

Cold sore attacks are also viral originated and are effectively treated with this protocol. Many over the counter topical remedies for cold sores have lysine as the active ingredient.

Lysine may reduce calcium loss in urine, which especially as an anti-aging therapy prevents the onset of osteoporosis. It may also retard the effects and begin the reversal of osteoporosis.

Best natural source: wheat germ, oat flakes.

Leucine, Isoleucine and Valine

These are branched chain amino acids. They are essential amino acids whose carbon structure is marked by a branch point, but have different metabolic routes. They act together metabolizing in the skeletal muscle and, to a lesser extent, the liver, and are some of the primary constituents of muscle tissue.

They promote protein synthesis or uptake. Leucine acts separately as a major metabolic regulator and serves as an alternative energy source for the body to glucose. It stimulates insulin release in muscle and other tissues, insulin not only stimulating protein synthesis but inhibiting protein breakdown.

As a group they work effectively in the treatment of liver disease in cirrhotic patients, including alcoholism related cirrhosis.

Stress brought on by starvation, injury, surgery or infection are all aided by supplementation of this amino acid group. Exercise requires additional intake to replenish levels depleted.

Best natural source: wheat germ, granola, oat flakes.

L-methionine

A very complicated contributor to the body's chemistry. Methionine performs three primary functions. As a methyl donor it combines with ATP (adenosine, triphosphate, an energy containing molecule) to form active methionine. This compound then contributes to the bio-synthesis of deanol, choline, serine, creatine, epinephrine and carnitine.

As a sulphur containing amino acid, methionine is a compound of pain relieving methionine, enkephalin, and various endorphins.

Methionine plays a critical role in the delicate balance of tissue repair, organ function, and the anabolic state of protein synthesis. Working in conjunction with folic acid, methionine is an allergy fighter of asthma and chronic pain.

Methionine is also used as an anti-depressant, and there are studies on its use in dermatology, urology, surgery, chronic pain and radiation therapy. Methionine requires more than just a cursory mention or brief description. In essence what it does in the body is contribute to the synthesis of many important compounds. It is also a principal ingredient of most good anti-oxidant formulas.

Best natural source: wheat germ.

L-threonine

Threonine breaks down in the body to glycine, serine and glucose and fuels the neurotransmitters, acetylcholine, serotonin, catecholamines and histamine.

Threonine is used in the treatment of depression: glycine acts as a sedative to the brain. As an immune stimulant, threonine promotes the growth of the thymus gland, the body's immune regulator.

Threonine is also a component in the body's anti-inflammatory complex, and because of its muscle relaxant properties is used in the treatment of spastic conditions.

Best natural source: wheat germ.

L-histidine

Another component of the body's anti-inflammatory complex. In rheumatoid arthritis patients, histidine shows up in low levels in the synovial fluid, the lubricating fluid secreted by the joints. If arthritis is an auto-immune disease, where the body attacks itself, we begin to see the deficiencies that facilitate this condition.

Histidine plays vital roles in the body's metabolic function and in repair of cell tissues damaged due to viruses, toxins or allergens. In the treatment of stress, histidine is needed more than any other amino acid.

Histidine is the parent molecule of histamine, which is stored throughout the body and is a major neurotransmitter in the brain. Histamine is stored in the blood platelets, mast cells and basophils. Basophils contain the most blood histamine which triggers the antibodies to regulate immune responses.

Histidine is also a contributor to the production of hydrochloric acid in the stomach and is associated with the facilitation of orgasms in both men and women through histamine.

Best natural source: wheat germ.

The non-essential amino acids are:

L-alanine

This is found in high concentrations in muscle, and is one of the most important amino acids released by muscle as a form of energy in the body. Alanine is quickly converted into glucose by the liver.

Hypoglycaemia can be treated by alanine, which stimulates an increase in blood sugar, triggering the release of the hormone glucagon. It has the same effect on diabetes: ketones (result of incomplete oxidation of fats), found in the blood of diabetics, are potent cross-linkers: alanine reduces elevated triglycerides which inhibit the breakdown of protein and the release of alanine from the liver.

Alanine may benefit immune deficient individuals through the role it plays in the lymphocytes. It also contributes to the growth of the thymus, the body's immune regulator.

Alanine also can play a significant role in breaking down kidney stones and in their prevention.

Best natural source: wheat germ.

L-arginine

Arginine is an amino acid of ammonia production, as ammonia is turned into urea in the liver. Its primary metabolic role is in the urea cycle, the biochemical pathway which metabolizes nitrogen and protein. Urea, the main nitrogen-containing constituent in urine, is the final product of protein metabolism. Arginine is essential to the transport, storage and excretion of nitrogen.

Liver injury and disorders (hepatic cirrhosis, fatty liver, etc.) result in ammonia intoxication because of the liver's impaired ability to metabolize urea. Arginine therapy can be successful if there is some natural reserve within the liver.

Arginine plays a vital role in the metabolism of protein because of its ability to transport, store and excrete nitrogen. Muscle growth is dependent on this process, and other compounds used in muscle derived from arginine: guanidophosphate, phosphoarginine, and creatine. Arginine enhances the utilization of glucose.

Arginine has been used clinically in the treatment of certain cancers, specifically in retarding tumours by reducing the chemical biosynthesis needed for tumour cell growth. Research indicates arginine may be thymus stimulating, preventing aging atrophy and promoting the maintenance of a healthy immune system.

Arginine is one of the principal catalysts in the body's production of collagen, the main support protein of skin tendons, bone, cartilage and connective tissue.

Best natural source: wheat germ.

L-asparagine and Aspartic Acid

Asparagine is synthesized by the body from aspartic acid and adenosine triphosphate (ATP). Aspartic acid is synthesized from glutamate, with vitamin B6 as a co-factor. This is very important example of how the body's chemistry laboratory produces various chemical reactions using its metabolic pathways to regulate its functions. Asparagine provides the brain with energy and regulates the central nervous system.

Aspartic acid is unique in terms of amino acids in that it plays two major roles in the metabolism of ammonia and of carbohydrates. It acts as a neurotransmitter in the brain for brain energy metabolism. Aspartic acid is a component in the formation of DNA.

Aspartic acid may be an immunostimulant of the thymus gland and protect against damage from radiation.

Best natural source: wheat germ.

L-carnitine

There is so much to say about this wonderful amino acid. It acts as a fat regulator, by carrying fat across the membrane into the energy burning mitochondria of each cell. The oxidized fat is stored as energy as adenosine triphosphate (ATP), the fuel for most of the body's mechanical functions such as muscle contraction.

It also helps the body oxidize amino acids, preventing the body from raiding muscle tissue or branched chain amino acids during prolonged exertion or exercise, when carbohydrates supplies have been exhausted. This is especially important to athletes, weight lifters, etc. who can easily defeat their efforts if the body draws from muscle rather than fat for fuel. Recovery time after exercise is improved with carnitine.

Carnitine regulates fat in the heart, a muscle, where one of the main sources of energy is fat and where the highest concentration is found in the body.

Carnitine can reduce ketone levels in the blood, which are the result of the incomplete oxidation of fats. Diabetics are especially subject to ketones, as are people with high fat diets.

Carnitine helps to provide sperm with mobile energy.

Dialysis patients lose most of their blood carnitine during treatment. Receiving carnitine after treatment can lessen the effects of muscle weakness and anaemia, and provide needed oxygen to body tissue.

For heart patients it also, besides metabolizing triglycerides fats, strengthens the heart, improving irregular beats and palpitations or arrhythmias. An excellent tonic for heart disease.

Carnitine is synthesized in the body from the amino acid lysine, which requires a multi-step process and the right combination of the following: the amino acid methionine, vitamins C and B, niacin, and the minerals, iron and manganese. This is indicative of the body's utilization of not only amino acids but also of vitamins, minerals, herbs, etc., where, unless the right catalysts are present or enzymatic action takes place, no benefit is received.

Best natural source: carnitine supplements 1,800–3,600 mg per day, broken up over the course of the day to 600–1,200 mg per time. (Needs lysine and methionine for synthesis.)

Gamma Aminobutyric Acid, Glutamic acid and Glutamine

This is an amazing combination of amino acids that work in unison to perform many functions from energy to the operation of brain reactions.

Glutamic acid (GA) is the spark plug or neurotransmitter of neurons in the nerves of the brain. GA is converted by the body into glutamine (GAM) and gamma-amino butyric acid (GABA).

GAM is a major fuel source for the brain and the entire body. GABA is an energy source which produces a tranquilizing effect on the brain with its inhibitory neurotransmitter properties. It also plays a role in the function of the pancreas, duodenum and the thymus.

These three amino acids work together creating a synergy that is extremely active in all brain functions: including fuel, the stimulant and sedative effects on the nervous system, the regulation of glands and organs, and the synthesis and metabolism of other chemical and compound reactions in the body.

GABA is probably the most therapeutic of the three, and it is used to treat hypertension and nervous disorders (epilepsy, spastic syndromes, etc.). It is also used as an appetite suppressant, and to reduce blood sugar levels in diabetics. It is important to remember that vitamin B6 and manganese are important in the conversion of GA to GABA.

GAM has been effective in the treatment of alcoholism, reducing the craving for sugar, since GAM provides adequate energy for the brain in the absence of the glucose produced by alcohol.

Monosodium glutumate (MSG) is the evil twin of GA. It is the sodium salt of glutamic acid and, because it is readily absorbed by the blood stream, is toxic at low levels. The usual symptoms are dizziness, headaches and abdominal cramps. Children especially are extremely susceptible to its adverse effects. Stay away from MSG. Always ask when in doubt if it is being used.

Best natural source: wheat germ.

L-glycine

Glycine is an important metabolic agent to the body. Some of its functions include the building up of glycogen levels (stored energy), and the manufacture of DNA, skin proteins, collagen, cholesterol conjugates, and the amino acid glutathionine.

Glycine passes the blood brain barrier and is one of three amino acids that act as inhibitory neurotransmitters in the brain. Glycine also acts as a sedative and has been effective in the treatment of depression, epilepsy and spastic related disorders.

Glycine funds the pituitary, important in regulating serum growth hormones and the repair of muscle fibres. Glycine in conjunction with arginine causes nitrogen to be retained in the body, allowing amino acids to be absorbed easier and speeding up wound healing. Glycine reduces uric acid in the system, important in the treatment of gout.

Best natural source: wheat germ.

L-ornithine

Ornithine releases a growth hormone that promotes tissue growth. It is converted into arginine by the body, both in its natural state and as a supplement. Ornithine in conjunction with carnitine metabolizes body fat. Ornithine's role in the body supports that of arginine, neutralizing ammonia, stabilizing amino acid imbalances, and improving liver function and the immune system.

Best natural source: wheat germ.

L-proline (and Hydroxy-L-proline)

Proline is produced by the body from glutamate or ornithine. Both are completely separate source pathways. Glutamate is linked to carbohydrate metabolism, and ornithine to protein metabolism, thus forming a unique metabolic bridge.

Hydroxyproline is produced from proline and is the principal constituent of collagen. Its primary role is in the production of bone and connective tissue. It is interesting to note that almost a third of the body's proteins are found in collagen. Collagen is the principal ingredient of cartilage, tendons, all connective tissue and the heart muscle. It literally is the glue that keeps the body's organs, bones and muscles in place.[13]

Best natural source: wheat germ.

L-serine

Serine is produced by the body from glycine and is concentrated in cell membranes. It contributes to the production of ethanolamine, choline, phospholipids and sarcosine. All of these are essential to form neuro-transmitters and stabilize cell membranes.

Serine has an important role in the body's chemistry laboratory, converting to glycine and then to amino levulinic acid (ALA), a precursor of haemoglobin. It is also metabolized to pyruvate (in Krebs cycle), which participates in glucose building. Serine serves to combine carbohydrates to form the glycoproteins that build structural proteins, i.e. hormones, enzymes.

Serine is produced from L-glycine in the body, and I would recommend this as the source for individual L-serine supplementation.

Best natural source: wheat germ.

L-taurine

While a non-essential amino acid, because the body can synthesize its own taurine, it is essential to pre-term/new born infants and is found in mothers' milk.

The body produces taurine from cysteine (with vitamin B6 present), but it has not been established if it produces enough. A question remains about the need for a dietary supplement of taurine.

Taurine is not found in the make-up of protein (muscle) but operates in the body as a free molecule. Even though it is a water soluble molecule and does not pass through the body's fatty membranes, it is in fact found in almost all membranes, the heart, white blood cells, the central nervous system and the brain. Taurine is also found in bile, where it binds to bile acids for the digestion of fats and the absorption of fat soluble vitamins.

Its principal roles are related to the brain, heart, gall bladder, eyes and vascular system. It transfers sodium, potassium, calcium and magnesium ions in and out of cells and is involved in the regulation of electrical charge on the cell membranes.

Taurine, next to GABA, is the most important inhibitory neurotransmitter in the brain, where it acts as an anti-convulsant/anti-anxiety agent.

Taurine also plays many important metabolic roles, stimulating prolactin and insulin release. It increases biliruben and cholesterol excretion in the bile, vital to gall bladder function. In the treatment of heart disease, i.e. congestive heart failure, post-myocardial infarction and pre-ventricular arrhythmia, taurine can be effective in doses of 500 mg to 5 g through oral supplementation. This treatment can also be used for epilepsy, gall stones, mitral valve prolapse, hypertension, retinitis pigmentosa (light sensitivity) and diabetes.

Overall taurine is a very important contributor to many of the body's operating systems. The amino acids alanine, glutamic acid and pantothenic acid inhibit taurine metabolism, while cysteine, and vitamin B6, produce it.

Best natural source: wheat germ.

Summary of amino acid requirements

Amino acids are what our body uses to produce protein. They make up the brain's neurotransmitters, liver and intestinal enzymes, along with all the enzyme systems of different cells.

Without these enzymes, there is no way we can either absorb vitamins and minerals, or fund the thousands of chemical reactions necessary daily.

In my anti-aging research, amino acid therapy is the corner stone to stopping the biological clock. A slow death begins when our body cannot produce the thousands of chemical reactions necessary to metabolize hormones, form muscles, connective tissue, and enzymes, and produce neurotransmitters.

Without this fountain of youth, atrophy and degeneration begin. Do yourself a favour, get a blood test and note your albumin reading. Albumin is an indicator of protein; globulin is manufactured primarily by the liver, which needs amino acids to produce globulin. (Globulin is a principal ingredient in the immune system.) Chances are you are deficient or, at worst, producing incomplete protein, which the immune system treats as a foreign invader.

Reflect back on and read more about the various roles that each amino acid plays. Understanding their interplay and their genetic and environmental deficiencies will provide not only the clues but the keys to unlocking the door of your individual body chemistry.

Supplementation

Don't be afraid to experiment. This is an exciting time because there are many great quality amino acids (free-form) on the market. Hopefully the FDA will not limit our freedom in the United States to purchase them over the counter, as they have threatened.

Keep in mind the protocol for taking free-form amino acids discussed earlier in this chapter. On an empty stomach, preferably first thing in the morning 30–60 minutes before your first meal. Take with a juice (simple carbohydrate), vitamin B6, and vitamin C. I take mine with a B-Complex which includes B6.

As mentioned throughout this chapter, the best natural source of amino acids is wheat germ. If you find it difficult to afford amino acid supplementation, wheat germ is relatively inexpensive. Look for vacuum packed wheat germ; this is important because wheat germ is highly unstable and oxidizes quickly if exposed to air. It can be mixed into a protein drink, or sprinkled on (preferably cold cereal). Keep it in a sealed container after opening and refrigerate.

Other complete sources of amino acids are wheat grass and bee pollen (but make sure you are not allergic to bees). The body instantly identifies with all three sources and begins processing and utilizing them immediately.

You will truly be amazed by the results of following an amino acid regimen.

7

Alcohol and Drugs

There is a network of slender gray cells which are circuitously stretched to form a column of narrow vertical sheets in the lower reaches of the brain, at about the point where you massage the top of your neck muscles below the skull. On their lower side they pick up sense nerves coming in from the body, and on their top side they send these impulses up to the higher reaches of the brain. All of our sense impulses go through this network. Because of the vast amount of input to the brain, the reticular formation decides what information is to be for special attention. It does this by adding to certain incoming signals additional signals which attract the attention of the higher brain centres the nerve impulses are going to meet. Acting as an intake censor, only those signals the reticular formation considers significant pass through to the awareness centre just behind the forehead.

These incredibly long, stretching cells that poke, weave and curl into almost all parts of the brain enable the reticular formation to ensure consciousness. In theory this seems a paradox, since the reticular formation is just a dumb net of cells. How does it decide which information is important enough to get through to the very top of the brain that has all of the reasoning power?

The body addresses this question by tagging all incoming signals. Nerve cells throughout the body are built to give their strongest message only when the impulse they are struck by is a changing one. In this way the reticular formation keeps us awake and ensures that attention is focused on the most important things. Otherwise, if the reticular formation passed on every incoming signal at the same time with equal emphasis to the high centres of the brain, we would be overwhelmed and in a constant state of exhausted consciousness. There are ways, however, in which the reticular formation is confused; the usual culprits being alcohol and drugs.

Alcohol

Everything we take into the body has an effect on its chemistry. Alcohol is one on those unique substances that can pass through the blood brain barrier, penetrating and affecting all aspects of the body's functions. It is amazing to think that alcohol can do this to an otherwise iron clad defence system. Proteins that are too big, minerals that are too 'sharp', are repulsed. But alcohol penetrates, like a stealth bomber; its molecules slip through totally undetected.

Let us begin with that first drink passing the lips. Alcohol is very effervescent, its molecules hurtling into the air. Inside the mouth it is no less subtle, bombarding the back of the throat and up the nose where the delicate taste receptors are. A small amount is absorbed into the bloodstream this way.

Once swallowed, the same bombarding alcohol molecules stimulate the mesh of blood vessels beneath the mucus surface of the stomach which are usually closed. The alcohol has now made them grow red and absorbent so that about 20% of the alcohol is ingested through the stomach lining. Food in the stomach at this point, especially food rich in fats and proteins, will absorb a lot of the alcohol.

The next port of call is the small intestine where the remaining 80% of absorption takes place. Then a direct path into the bloodstream, where the small capillary laden villi of the small intestine readily absorb the alcohol. From here it takes a mainline through the hepatic portal vein gateway, just under the ribs, directly into the liver. Initially the liver converts about $\frac{1}{200}$ of an ounce of alcohol molecules each minute (by a series of versions from alcohol molecule to super molecule) to a substance which the body can utilize as food for muscle, fat, or bone. This conversion takes place in fractions of a second and is facilitated through enzymes present in the liver.

So far so good; but once the $\frac{1}{200}$ of an ounce has been exceeded, which is almost instantly, the liver has no more space to process alcohol in its oblong chambers. The alcohol instead is sent in its pure untreated form into the blood stream where it is pumped to every organ of the body, including (as discussed earlier) through the blood brain barrier directly into the brain.

The brain utilizes almost 20% of the body's available oxygen, a supply which must be constant because the brain has no ability to store oxygen. Alcohol, however, consumes oxygen like a Pac-man in the bloodstream. Once past the cortex it enters the reticular formation. The bombarding alcohol molecules begin confusing and short-circuiting the reticular formation, dulling the brain's ability to react to or register many sensations that would otherwise not escape. A brief alcohol effect study would be the following:

(grams/ml)	The reticular formation is now performing at half
0.03–0.05	capacity in terms of incoming information being tagged for attention.
0.05–0.07	Fatty membrane of brain cells are penetrated,

	hand-eye reflexes begin slowing, driving ability is impaired.
0.09–0.10	The area controlling motor control, the pre-frontal region where the nerves controlling willed movement start from, is now affected. The alcohol molecules in their frenzy confuse the nerves, transmitting garbled messages down the nerve paths all the way to the end of muscles; limbs become wobbly, balance is affected. Hearing is dulled as alcohol molecules bounce against the inner ear's delicate nerves.
0.12–0.15	Staggering and intoxication.
0.30	Coma.
0.60	Death.

Now the after effects. Depending on the level of inebriation, you are most likely guaranteed a headache, due to the change in the balance of electrically charged particles in the blood and brain. You are definitely thirsty, because alcohol alters the body's precise arrangement of fluids, divided at 67% in the cells, and 25% between tissues and the rest in the blood – the brain for example is 85% water. Alcohol short-circuits the delicate filtration and absorption of the kidneys, telling it to send out much more fluid through the bladder than normal. And the severity of your hangover is intensified by the toxic side effects of the additives used in the manufacture of liquor. These include flavouring agents, sugar, dyes, molecule cleaning agents, ethers, alums, aldehydes and lime sulphate.

Alcohol depletes all available C and B vitamins from the blood stream. These water soluble vitamins are vital substances required for many fundamental processes in the body, most importantly as electron transporter in many enzymatic reactions. This short-circuits the body's ability to communicate and provide damage control. The impact on the body is substantial: impaired is the ability to detoxify free radicals, anti-bacterial and anti-viral function, and the immune system is debilitated.

Things to do to neutralize and re-stabilize the body's chemistry from the effects of alcohol are:

1. Recent research presented at the Third Conference on Vitamin C found that vitamin C oxidizes alcohol. It does this by producing a peroxide which is then used by catalase in the oxidation of alcohol. Vitamin C is also the constituent (ascorbate) of the body's detoxification system, helping to speed up the elimination of alcohol. It also reduces fat accumulation in the liver caused by alcohol.

2. Alcohol pulls water from the body; but as it takes water from the

cells, the body sets up an alarm which triggers a release of chemicals that attempt to soak water back into the cells. Receptors, especially those in the mouth, become very sensitive, and the thirst level is extremely high as the body attempts to stabilize itself. Distilled water at room temperature is the preferred source.

3. Alcohol destroys oxygen molecules as well as playing havoc with the delicate balance of the brain's chemistry. The combination is a throbbing headache or hangover. An oxygenator will come in very handy, i.e. wheat grass, to stabilize the brain and reduce pain.

Drugs

Through their stealth shaped molecules, drugs, like alcohol, not only get through the reticular formation but also scramble it in the process. Hallucinogens like LSD, heroin, cocaine and amyl nitrate and drugs like amphetamines, nicotine and caffeine stimulate the reticular formation in a manner it was not designed to sustain.

Nerves that have received no signal from the body sense receptors confuse the reticular formation into thinking that there is significant chemical activity. The brain cannot disprove this non-existent activity, and opens gates that would not under normal conditions be accessible. The reticular formation, with its incredible screening process of information, is now on 'random access'; and thought, memory, sensation, etc. are now impaired by whatever chemical inducement is involved.

Many chemical drugs are addictive because they block the transmission of signals between certain brain cells. This makes the nerves much less sensitive to the natural chemicals that connect them and help to carry the signals. As a result feelings of anxiety, depression, pain, etc. are short-circuited and suppressed.

As the effects of the drugs wear off, the brain, which has adapted to this altered state, now returns to a state of heightened sensitivity and awareness. Whatever you were feeling before is now amplified, and addiction begins as one tries to recover that altered state.

8

Cell Salts

The Twelve Tissue Salts

Blood salts, tissue salts, call them what you will, are the constituents of tissue building that play a vital role in the body's chemistry. There are twelve tissue salts found in the blood,[14] as determined by Dr Schussler of Germany in a paper published in 1873 based on research started in the 1830s by Samuel Hahnemann. Hahnemann pioneered homeopathy; but Schussler ascertained that cell salts enacted the physiologico-chemical processes that took place within an organism and were not based on homeopathic laws of cure.

If there are twelve salts that float around in the blood, what role do they play? Schussler determined that there are two kinds of substance needed in the tissue building process, organic and inorganic constituents. Organic substances are sugar, fat and albuminous material, which serve as the physical basis of tissue. Water and salts, like potash, lime, silica, iron, magnesium, and sodium, are the inorganic substances that determine the particular kind of cell to be built up.

For the body to function as the incredible chemistry laboratory it is, all the raw materials must be present. Some people are genetically deficient in cell salts, others are deficient because of dietary or environmental causes. Once you realize how vital cell salts are to healthy cells and tissue building, it becomes obvious that deficiencies can form a 'domino' effect, of producing incomplete, dysfunctional cells which make the body vulnerable to disease.

I advise most people to supplement with a good cell salt formula that includes the twelve bioplasmic constituents. These form the inorganic materials that help form muscles, nerve, brain and connective tissue, and break down as follows:

Nerve cells –	Magnesia Phos, Kali Phos, Natrum and Ferrum
Muscle cells –	Magnesia Phos, Kali Phos, Natrum, Ferrum and Kali Mur
Connective tissue –	Silica (Elastic Tissue contains Calcarea Fluor)

Bone cells –	Calcarea Fluor, Magnesia Phos and large amounts of Calcarea Phos
Cartilage & mucous cells –	Natrum Mur
Hair and eyes –	Natrum Mur and Ferrum

These inorganic materials combine with all the organic components carried in the blood, oxygen being a principal catalyst to form an alchemy of chemical affinities. The result is new individual cells that make up the various tissue of muscle, nerve, brain, bone, and connective tissue, along with mucous membrane and hair.

The quality of the cells our body produces is directly related to the quality and availability of the ingredients available. If you were born with a deficiency in a particular cell salt or if because of dietary or environmental reasons there is an imbalance, this deficiency will manifest itself in your body and will be unique to you and your particular chemistry. This can involve diseases and disorders too numerous to mention. Because these minute inorganic salts play such an important role in understanding our body's chemistry, I suggest reviewing the twelve cell salts individually, in terms of their specific contributions. You can then look at your own body, compare conditions with any you may be experiencing, and discover a lack of any particular salt(s).

Genetic weaknesses are sometimes best described as an incomplete chemical reaction in which the mutation, as it continues to reproduce itself, becomes the norm, affecting a particular aspect of the body's function. In diseased cells this chemical mutation has progressed to a point where it is deleterious to the body. A good example to reflect on in terms of understanding the significant role cell salts play is Chapter 10 on electrolytes. Without the minerals in constant supply our body could not maintain the electrical charge necessary to sustain life.

Biochemical cell salts are administered in minimal doses in direct correlation to the minuteness to the cellular salts found in the tissues. It is in this diluted, derivative state that they can enter the blood and intercellular fluids. This is accomplished by sublingual (under the tongue) absorption, a direct pathway into the bloodstream. It is very important to stress just how important it is that the salts are diluted to a size whereby the molecules can be absorbed in the oral cavity. Anything larger gets passed on to the stomach where it is converted into something else. For example with iron, if in trying to absorb ferrous phosphate (the cell salt) it reaches the stomach, it is converted to a chloride.

Many mineral waters (as discussed earlier) contain inorganic salts, but unfortunately in a molecular size that renders them unusable by the cells. In fact their size makes them a liability, because the body tries to expel what it cannot absorb, which is not an easy task. Certain mineral springs whose waters have been hailed as curative owe this to the fact that the minerals are in a diluted enough state to allow uptake by the body through the skin.

Biochemical cell salts or their molecules when made available to the cells correct disturbed molecular motion (as described by Schussler), wherein the molecular rotation through deficiencies can be altered or disturbed, thus causing disease. These cell salt constituents, directly administered as homogeneous like substances, can reprogramme the cells back to health. It is interesting to note at this point that homeopathic remedies act indirectly, and conversely are administered as heterogeneous unlike substances to the cells.

Tissue remedies of cell salts are prepared like all homeopathic remedies, according to the decimal or centisimal scale in trituration (preparing into a fine powder) or dilution. We are talking about minute dosages, infinitesimal grains of a salt administered in a highly diluted or homeopathic form. This really is the theory of 'less is more', since the molecular size of the triturated salt is such that it can readily enter the bloodstream. This re-establishes normal cell equilibrium since these infinitesimal doses correspond to the minuteness of the cellular salts in the tissues.

The dosages most common are as follows: 3X, 6X, 12X, 30X, 1M, 10M, CM

1X = 0.10 gram of crude substance or 1/10

1C = 0.01 gram of crude substance or 1/100

1C = 2X

6C = 12X

1M = 1000C

10M = 10,000C

$\frac{1}{100}$ or 1C trituration of a salt is estimated to contain 16 trillion molecules, which more than illustrates the power these minute dosages have to restore disturbed molecular rotation back to equilibrium. Smaller dosages are recommended for a 'rapid, gentle and permanent restoration of health', according to Dr Hahnemann.

The Twelve Tissue Salts are:

Calcarea Fluorica (Calc. Fluor) (Fluoride of Lime)

Properties – Found in the surface of bones and enamel of teeth, constituent of elastic fibres and epidermis (skin, connective tissue, vascular walls).

Remedies – Diseases of blood and blood vessels, including remedy for varicose and enlarged veins. Auto-immune disorders where joints, cartilage, synovial membrane, and connective tissue are affected, i.e. arthritis, tennis elbow, chronic synovitis (joint inflammation), fibroid tumours, and exostoses (tumours of bone, benign) i.e. lumps on skin.

Calcarea Phosphorica (Calc. Phos) (Phosphate of Lime)

Properties – Essential to proper growth and nutrition of body. Found in blood plasma, saliva, gastric fluids, bones, connective tissue, and teeth. Initiates cell growth, an important constituent of alliumin and nutrient transport and the coagulation of blood.

Remedies – All bone diseases, gout, rheumatic and arthritic conditions. Immune system stimulant, reverses anaemia by building haemoglobin (red blood cells) and regulating discharges of lymph system, mucous membranes, and glands.

Calcarea Sulphurica (Calc. Sulph) (Gypsum)

Properties – Works in the liver destroying worn out red blood cells, by removing their water. This prevents a build-up of dead red blood cells in the spleen and provides efficient removal through the bile.

Remedies – Reduces swelling and discharge of mucous membranes, skin eruptions, ulcers and abscesses of the intestinal tract. Inflammation of connective tissue and lymphatic glands. Most if not all ulcerations with discharge (boils, acne, cysts etc.).

Ferrum Phosphoricum (Ferr. Phos) (Phosphate of Iron)

Properties – Iron is what gives haemoglobin or red blood cells their colour. Iron also attracts oxygen, carrying it through the blood stream and with the interaction of Kali. Sulph. into individual cells. A molecular disturbance in the equilibrium of iron in muscle fibres causes them to relax. In the blood vessels this causes dilation and increases blood pressure. In the intestinal tract the villi and peristaltic action relax causing diarrhoea. Its ability to attract and carry oxygen into the muscle prevents this from happening. An important catalyst for enzymatic action, vitamin C can increase absorption by 30%. Iron is also vital for healthy immune function, cellular respiration and peroxide deactivation. It is also required for the production of a number of proteins, haemoglobin, myoglobun, and cytochrome.

Remedies – Treatment of anaemia, loss of energy and strength. It also regulates bowels and reduces inflammations. Do not supplement during infection, as bacteria use iron to grow; but the body will not release its stored iron during this time.

Kali Mureaticum (Kali. Mur) (Potassium Chloride)

Properties – Responsible for new brain cell formation. Found in blood corpuscles, muscles, nerve and brain cells, as well as intercellular fluids. It is similar to and shares many of the same properties of sodium chloride, such as stimulating the uptake of glucose and fluid in the small intestine, and stabilizing extracellular fluid volume.

Remedies – Used in the treatment of swelling and inflammation of the mucous membranes, lymph gland, and the small gaps (interstitial) between the connective tissue. Effective in treating sodium-induced hypertension and stabilizing blood pressure. Joint stiffness and rheumatic conditions, i.e. gout and swelling around the joints and the pain associated with these conditions, can be aided especially by the triturations and dilution of this particular cell salt.

Kali Phosphoricum (Kali. Phos) (Phosphate of Potash)

Properties – A constituent of all fluids and tissues, especially those of the brain, nerve, muscle, and blood cells. Funds chemical reactions that rely on its alkaline ability to prevent free radical oxidation from fat and chemical pollutants. Important in the formation and maintenance of brain, nerve and muscle tissue. Has astringent antiseptic properties.

Remedies – Used in the treatment of all nerve disorders – neurogenic (nervous origin, neuralgia, or neurasthenia), cerebral anaemia, aging and atrophied conditions, and septic (bacterial) infections.

Kali Sulphurican (Kali. Sulph) (Potassium Sulphate)

Properties – Acts with the oxide of iron as an oxygen carrier. Found in the cells and intercellular fluids, muscles, nerves, epithelium, and red blood cells.

Remedies – Treatment of skin disorders, repairing and replacing epidermis (outer skin layer) and epithelium (tissue composing tissue/skin), making up respiratory, digestive and urinary systems. Treatment of discharges from mucous membranes. Conditions attributed to free radical oxidation of cells.

Magnesium Phosphorica (Magnes. Phos) Phosphate of Magnesia

Properties – Constituent of muscles, nerves, bone, brain, spine, teeth and red blood cells. Magnesium is vital to enzymatic action and is a catalyst in calcium and potassium uptake. Helps to form bone and facilitate carbohydrate and mineral metabolism. Important constituent in maintaining the body's electrolyte balance.

Remedies – Treatment for nerve disorders, nerve and muscle impulse transmission where symptoms are anxiety, nervousness or irritability. Effective for depression, muscle cramping or spasms. Important in the treatment of high blood pressure and heart disease.

Natum Muriaticum (Natr. Mur) (Sodium Chloride)

Properties – Sodium (the regulator of body fluids and water in cells) is pumped out of the cell and forms its protective membrane. Each cell has a sodium pump removing sodium from the cell and leaving potassium in. One of the most important substances in blood plasma (which is the fluid of blood, minus red and white cells). Body maintains approximately 11 ounces of sodium to regulate body functions. This salt not only regulates moisture within the cells, it attracts water molecules from the blood stream into the cells, prompting cell division. If this equilibrium is disturbed by lack of sodium in the cells, water is retained in the intercellular fluids (tissue); causing hydraemia (excessive fluid content of the blood), bloating and fatigue. Excessive sodium in the intercellular fluids causes acrid odour from perspiration and discharge from mucous membranes into the intestinal tract, causing diarrhoea. Sodium of the Natr. Mur molecules in the peptic (digestive) glands spins off chloride which unites with hydrogen to form the only acid the body produces, hydrochloric acid, used in the stomach to initially break down food.

Remedies – Because of trituration, Natr. Mur is much more active and available to the cells than regular salt. This allows the cells to immediately start absorbing water (in dehydrated cells and tissue) or eliminating excesses of fluid from too much sodium. Sodium is used in the regulation of hypertension, anaemia, kidney, and liver diseases. Because sodium is critical to so many body functions – being an electrolyte in the blood, it maintains blood pressure, acid-base balance, nerve and muscle function and digestive fluids – it is almost impossible to talk about a condition in the body where Natr. Mur would not play a healing role.

Natrum Phosphoricum (Natr. Phos) (Sodium Phosphate)

Properties – Found in the blood, muscles, nerve and brain cells, and intercellular fluids. Glycogen provides muscles with energy and produces lactic acid; Natr. Phos converts lactic acid into carbonic acid and water, which it absorbs and carries through the blood stream to the lungs where it is exchanged by oxygen for carbon dioxide. Natr. Phos prevents lactic acid from building up in the blood, and uric acid; both form crystals that attack the mucous membrane and soft tissue when their levels are elevated. Natr. Phos serves to break down or emulsify acids, carrying them from the intestinal wall into the blood and finally to the tissues.

Remedies – Apart from its preventative qualities, Natr. Phos reverses the effects of auto-immune disorders such as gastric ulcers, rheumatoid arthritis, gout, eczema, and lymphatic swelling.

Natrum Sulphuricum (Natr. Sulph)
(Sodium Sulphate)

Properties – Appears not in the cells but in the intercellular fluids. It neutralizes sulphuric acid formed by oxidation of protein (albuminoids) that would destroy tissues. Natr. Sulph attracts water to eliminate worn out leucocytes (white blood cells). It triggers the release of fluid waste through the respiratory and digestive passages to the kidneys to be eliminated through the urinary tract. It also stimulates the sensory nerves of the bladder to control elimination, and the secretion of the bile ducts, pancreas, and intestinal tract.

Remedies – Because of its stimulant, cathartic (laxative) qualities, it is effective in the treatment of all respiratory, digestive and urinary tract disorders. Some of these would include diabetes, gout, gall bladder (stones), kidney stones, hydraemia (excessive fluid in the blood), oedema (excessive fluid in tissues), and catarrh (excessive secretion of mucous).

Silicea (Silica) (Silicic Oxide)

Properties – Found in the body as a (collagen forming) constituent of all connective tissue, joints, cartilage, ligaments, tendons, glands, skin and mucous surfaces. It is also found in hair, nails, and connective tissue of nerve fibres.

Remedies – Used to treat conditions affecting bones, joints, glands, skin and mucous surfaces. Silica can break down and re-absorb keloid (scar tissue), abscesses, and gout, which attack connective tissue at the joints. It also breaks down and absorbs bruises, boils, all suppurative (pus forming) eruptions, and, as with all these conditions, uses the lymphatic system to eliminate the irritants. Used to treat nervous system disorders (neuralgia) and cold sensitivities.

Summary

The alchemy that cell salts produce in the body provide the very foundation of all structure. Each cell salt and its individual properties will help you to fine tune your body's chemistry wherever it may be lacking; and by making the twelve salts (sold combined as *Bioplasma*) part of your daily regime will fortify your whole body.

9

Homeopathy

The 'law of similars' states that the same substance promoting a set of symptoms can in small quantities help a sick person with those symptoms get better.

As we discovered in Chapter 8 on cell salts, biochemistry is accomplished through the administration of homogenous (like) substances, whereas homeopathy is the indirect administration of heterogeneous (unlike) substances. Samuel Hahnemann, the founder of homeopathy, based his theory on the premise that a remedy can cure a disease if it produces symptoms similar to those of the disease in healthy organisms.

Homeopathy treats the individual, not the disease. By using the voluminous *Materia Medica*,[15] (the homeopathic handbook, written by Dr William Boericke, and originally published in 1927), it is possible to match a particular constitution and condition with the remedy to correct the imbalance. The allopathic physician is trained to categorize symptoms as conditions or specific diseases; to look at an individual's symptoms and try to determine what is causing them; then to find a substance in nature that, while organically different, can produce the same symptom in the body. The principle being that the substance, either plant, mineral, or animal, will stimulate the body's immune system into action. This theory, the same as applied to cell salts, is called positive and negative matching.

Most pharmaceutical medicines prescribed today treat symptoms and not the cause. For example, if you peel an onion, your eyes burn, itch and tear. Your nose may become runny and you may start sneezing, as with a cold. Taking a homeopathic dose of albium cepa (red onion) during a cold would stimulate your immune system to heal the aggravation. The pharmaceutical alternative would be a synthetic ephedrine, or a product that does a great job of masking the symptom but nothing in terms of stimulating the body's healing ability. If anything, these synthetic compounds create additional adverse chemical aggravations in the body.

When you find a condition or symptom with the corresponding remedy in the *Materia Medica* you are looking at a compendium of 200 years of research. The research consists of *in vitro* (laboratory) evidence and provings (human test subjects) which have established the efficacy of each individual remedy. Most provings involve numerous tests.

Homeopathic remedies come in pellet form like the cell salt pellets.[16] These are typically lactose and/or milk sugar, and hold the homeopathic substance in a neutral environment. The pellets are highly unstable and anything may contaminate them, such as touch by hands or chemicals. It is important when taking them to make sure that you do not handle them. Pour them into the lid of the bottle and drop them under your tongue. You may wish to alternate this method with taking a few pellets, dissolving them into a tablespoon of distilled water, and holding the solution in the mouth for 30–60 seconds. The latter method spreads the remedy throughout the oral cavity, triggering tongue innervation by a gentle shock to the nervous system.

Tinctures are another application, where the remedy has been combined with alcohol or distilled water. The same protocol applies in terms of not contaminating the solution; placing the drops in the oral cavity having not drunk anything for at least 15–30 minutes before or after, and taking them on an empty stomach.

The third application is topical, where the remedy has been added to a gel or an inert base. Here the application requires that the skin to which the remedy is applied is clean.

The dosage for the pellets or tinctures is the same formula as described for cell salts. A 'mother tincture' is created from the natural base substance (plant, mineral or animal) and alcohol or distilled water. The mother tincture is then diluted according to the decimal (X) or centisimal (C) scale. X potencies are diluted by using one part of mother tincture and 9 parts alcohol or water. Each time it is diluted it is vigorously shaken, causing molecular agitation, called potentization. As the dilution continues, 1 part substance to 9 parts solution or lactose, we obtain 2X, 3X, and so on. One C is one part substance and 99 parts alcohol or water, 2C is one part previous solution, 99 parts alcohol or water, etc. 1C is equal to 2X, 6C = 12X; thus you begin to understand the geometrics of the dilution and dosages.

Mega dosages are typically prescribed for chronic or acute diseases and should only be considered under a homeopath's care. These include dosages of 1M equal to 1,000C, 10M = 10,000C, CM = 100,000C, MM = 1,000,000C. Unless prescribed correctly, these can create homeopathic aggravation, as with mega doses of medication.

Hahnemann wrote: 'To get a prompt, gentle, lasting improvement, you most often need to use infinitesimal doses'. In this way the body receives only the amount it needs of a particular 'homeo' substance to correct an imbalance or 'pathos' (disease or suffering).

Become familiar with homeopathy. These biochemical minute substances, just as is the case with biochemical cell salts, are molecularly active and of a size that have the greatest effect on cells. The most powerful argument for biochemical and homeopathic remedies is that they are almost instantly available to the cells. Unlike all other nutrients, they require no conversion by the body to assimilate them or activate their properties. This approach to the body on a cellular level is one of the most powerful tools at our disposal for reprogramming our bodies for health.

Become familiar with this subtle science of less is more. Start looking at symptoms as markers or indicators to guide you to the problem, instead of reaching for remedies that treat the symptom.

Appendix A gives a recommendation of remedies that you may want to have on hand in your personal first aid kit as ready cures for the most common complaints. All of these are available at any good health food store or homeopathic pharmacy. Do yourself a favour and pick up a copy of a homeopathic *Materia Medica*, an excellent compendium giving you a range of over 700 remedies.

Remember that homeopathic remedies work through slow and gentle healing, primarily aimed at the cause not the symptom. Used properly they can prevent the onset of symptoms. This is difficult to impart, given the fact that we are so conditioned to reaching for remedies that neutralize the symptoms. So be patient, use homeopathy as preventative care and maintenance as well as to address problems when they arise.

10

Electrolytes

'Blood is Life' and pure blood can only come from good nutrients, which must be broken down through digestion in order to be carried not only into the blood stream but become constituents of the blood that feed the cells throughout the entire body.

If we look at the body as a chemistry laboratory, it defies in many ways all laws of chemical affinity and chemical proportion. In this century science re-discovered what was previously called 'Vital Life Force' as electrolytes or the body's electricity. In his book *Elements of Physiology*, Professor Muller describes how in chemistry certain elements combine in fixed proportions.[17] In organic bodies these elements were not only counteracted but formed combinations that were in direct opposition and defy chemical laws. Electrolytes create this chemical alchemy in the body, the life force, the electricity.

Electrolytes are made from dissolved minerals found in the blood that dissociate into charged particles, called ions. These negative and positive charged ions produce an electrical charge, like a battery.

Blood is the source from which life force draws all of its resources. From this one source each cell takes what it needs to maintain and repair all muscle, skin, tendon, brain tissue, bone, hair, etc. Conversely, poisons and toxins that find their way into the bloodstream produce the reverse effect, creating free radicals by destroying the cell.

As we look at the blood, we come upon the life force, electricity. The electricity the body produces is called electrolytes, made from dissolved minerals found in the blood that dissociate into charged particles, called ions. These create an electric charge, like a battery. The human body is like a machine that runs on positive and negative ions, without electrolytes and the electricity they produce, life is impossible.

Electrolytes maintain the acid/alkaline balance of the blood by their buffering action. They regulate blood volume and pressure throughout the body. Electrolytes also act as a carrying agent for certain amino acids and minerals. Everything involving electrolytes relates to balance necessary for the body to function properly.

If the mineral constituents of either negative or positive ions are out of balance, the body will develop immediate symptoms. These symptoms can include changes in blood pressure, muscle tension, fatigue, heat stroke, headaches. Severe imbalances or electrolyte loss can cause sudden death through heart failure. The mineral elements need to be in balance for the system to function. Typically this means that the anions and cations contain the same number of MEGS (mEg/L = milliquivalents per litre).

Cations and Anions

Negative ions are known as anions, while positive ions are cations. The minerals necessary to form these ions include the following cations:

Sodium (Na^+)
Potassium (K^+)
Calcium (Ca^{++})
Magnesium (Mg^{++})
And the following anions:
Chloride (Cl^-)
Bicarbonate (HCO_{3-})
Phosphate (HPO_{4--})

We lose electrolytes through daily activity, perspiration, exercise, etc., which need to be constantly replaced to keep our internal batteries charged. They also form an information superhighway, providing the current for the language the body uses to communicate with itself.

From a functional standpoint, for example, they provide the electricity to the cellular membrane, which separates the intracellular and extracellular compartments, to allow for the free movement of water molecules in and out of the cell. Sodium is pumped out of the cell and potassium is kept in; but if levels are out of alignment, and more sodium is ingested than potassium, the sodium pump slows down, causing the calcium pump also to slow down. As calcium builds up in the cells it increases the muscle tension of the blood vessel walls which increases blood pressure and causes fatigue. Remember that one-third of the body's energy is required just to pump sodium out, and potassium into the cells to make the electrical gradient.

If electrolytes permit the free flow of water molecules in and out of the cells, how much water do we need to be drinking? Two to three litres a day. A small percentage can come from fruits and vegetables, which are typically 90% water, but the majority needs to be water, preferably distilled with electrolytes added. Any time we are in a situation where we run the risk of losing body fluid, always remember that without water there is no life.

How much water is too much or too little?

Too much water can actually cause water intoxication, where the blood plasma expands the blood volume and the blood pressure, forcing abnormal amounts of water into the cells. This causes bloating and oedema (a condition many people can relate to when they have felt or been told that they are retaining water).

Dehydration, on the other hand, increases protein concentration in blood plasma, by taking water and potassium out of the cell. If serum potassium levels reach a dangerous level, the heart, which requires a lot of potassium, can develop an arrhythmia and stop beating.

The effects of an excess or deficiency of water are not necessarily so dramatic. A slow and constant auto-intoxication can over time cause havoc with body functions: waste products are not expelled, but re-circulate in the blood back to the cells; the circulatory system becomes constricted, with less oxygen available causing fatigue. And the brain, which requires a lot of water to provide the cushion it rests in, as with the ears and eyes which require water to transmit sound and light waves, can become unbalanced when blood flow is restricted due to dehydration. (Refer back to Chapter 5 on iridology: the area we described as the lymphatic rosary was created from a lack of water to flush out the lymph system.)

How to test for a deficiency of water

Cars have a dip stick to test fluid levels and here is an equivalent for the body. In a seated position, place your hand palm down on your thigh. You will or should begin to notice the veins on the back of your hand become slightly raised and puffy. Once your veins are firm and full of blood, slowly raise your arm up. If by the time they are at nipple level they are flat again, you are approximately a quart of fluid down.[18] If by chin level they are flat, you are a pint down. If your veins do not fill and raise in the resting position on the thigh, you are extremely low on fluid and your electrolytes are out of balance.

Remember that soft drinks, coffee and tea, with artificial sugars, phosphates, and caffeine, act as a diuretic, as does alcohol, stimulating the kidneys to release too much fluid from the body and with it important nutrients, the same nutrients that can be diluted due to too much water in the system. Balance is everything. (Refer back to Chapter 3 on digestion on this last point: see how the same thing happens when you consume too much liquid with a meal which dilutes the digestive enzymes and hydrochloric acid, preventing the nutrients from being broken down to a molecular form the body can assimilate.)

The more we know about symptoms and diseases the more we find that nutrition, and specifically the chemical imbalances in the blood and tissues, are at the root of our problems. This is why an appreciation of electrolytes lies at the beginning of an understanding of our unique biochemical individuality. Even genetically our genes determine the chromosomes, and chromosomes are responsible for the presence and efficiency of the body's enzyme system. Enzymes need the electrical charge produced by the dissolved minerals in every cell to allow them to function (glucose is also required as the fuel in the cell).

11

Free Radicals

If electrolytes are the spark of life, then free radicals are life's nemesis. Trying to find an example to explain this, I thought of the earth. If we look at the earth as the living breathing organism nature created, we realize that a lot has changed since the Garden of Eden. As the earth has aged, the effects of man have been profound: a world population that is doubling every thirty years, depleted natural resources, devitalized soil, and worst of all, pollution. These are the earth's free radicals.

So how do we equate earth pollution with free radical damage in the body?

The destruction of oxygen

Studies have shown that farming has gone from being environmentally friendly to destructive. Farmers across the United States use nitrogen fertilizer to grow grains. Because the soil lacks nitrogen from being constantly farmed, the only way to produce any kind of yield requires fertilizer. But only about 17–20% of the nitrogen stays in the soil to be utilized by the plant. The remaining nitrogen evaporates into the atmosphere.

Winds carry the nitrogen-laden air into metropolitan areas where it mixes with pollution, carbon gases from industry, car exhaust, fumes, etc. Any available oxygen binds to the nitrogen, which consumes it like a starving man; and sunshine oxidizes the nitrogen into nitrates and nitrites, which settle over cities as heavy molecules, preventing the penetration of free oxygen-laden air. This is why unhealthy air or smog is so harmful to all the living things that require oxygen for life.

Rain then washes the nitrates back into the soil, turning it alkaline and perpetuating the need for more fertilizer. These nitrates now appear in our food supply, not only devitalizing but also poisoning it. Our water becomes contaminated in this process – another large contributor to ground water pollution being nitrates from cattle manure. So if these are the free radicals destroying the earth's living organism, how do they act on the body?

A free radical is a molecular fragment, with one or more unpaired electrons, capable of damaging the cells, producing genetic damage and perhaps, cancer. It is a silent killer of cells that every day attacks the body, not only from external sources but also from internally produced chemical reactions. The three most known free radicals are the super oxide, the hydroxyl, and the peroxide. Created from toxins, radiation, carcinogens, stress, etc., this free orbiting molecule looks to join another molecule, typically a healthy cell, and share its electrons. This usually causes a chain reaction, turning healthy cells into more damaged free radical cells. By destroying the healthy cells, the free radicals, which are mutagens (cause mutations) and carcinogens (cause cancer), damage the DNA, and go on to produce even more destroyed cells or free radicals.

The body produces enzymes like super oxide dismutase (SOD) and glutathione peroxidase to prevent free radicals from coursing through the body creating havoc. But with the bombardment the body faces each day from free radicals caused by pollutants in the air, water, soil, food, chemical additives, smoking, alcohol, X-rays, etc., our free radical control systems are totally overwhelmed.

Our control systems of free radicals cause the body to produce the enzymes to destroy or neutralize free radicals in quantities typically proportional to the need, but this becomes a daunting task given the free radical exposure and the fact that most of us lack the raw materials necessary for our body to keep up a sustained offensive.

When the balance shifts and free radicals dominate our control systems the results are immune suppressant related conditions: cardiovascular disease, auto-immune disorders like arthritis, and cancer.[19] Over 100 conditions have been implicated to free radicals.

As the free radicals attack fatty acids in the body causing them to become peroxidized (rancid), they in turn become mutagens, carcinogens and immune suppressant free radicals.

In order for the body to do battle with the millions of free radicals we are exposed to daily, we need to produce a free radical fighting arsenal.[20] The body, as noted, mobilizes the arsenal of super oxide dismutase (SOD),[21] glutathione peroxidase, catalase and methionine reductase, formed from other anti-oxidant nutrients such as vitamin A, C, E, B1, B5, B6, PABA, Coenzyme CoQ^{10}, selenium, cysteine, and zinc. In addition, the following protocols also should be adopted.

Food:

Stay away from processed (hydrogenized polyunsaturated) or refined oils of any kind.[22] These oils oxidize (go rancid) very quickly once exposed to oxygen. Most packaged snacks, salad oils (other than olive oil) are very unstable; in fact use the rule of thumb that oils, nuts, grains, or any food stuffs that have an oil base are most likely oxidized unless they have been vacuum packed or freshly made.

Meats left exposed are very quickly subject to peroxidation, and carcinogens like bacteria grow very quickly. (We have seen cases of food poisoning in recent years become more prevalent, such as the E. coli bacteria outbreak in the *Jack in the Box* fast food chain referred to in Chapter 4.) Cooked foods, meat or anything that has been grilled or cooked to the point that it has char burned edges or surfaces are also very carcinogenic, full of free radical forming nitrates and nitrites. As Kedar Prasad Ph.D. states: 'Nitrosamines which result from the nitrosation of food constituents by ingested nitrites or nitrates, are one of the most potent human carcinogens'.

The largest source of nitrite intake in the USA is from cured meats, with cigarette smoke being the largest source of direct exposure to nitrosamines. Nitrates combine with haemoglobin to prevent the transport of oxygen to the cells causing fatigue, poor circulation and headaches. Nitrosamines are formed when nitrates combine in the stomach with protein. By irritating the complete digestive tract they enter the body, damaging the cells' DNA and turning them cancerous.

These dietary free radicals caused by peroxidized fats and oils are very carcinogenic: avoid them at all costs. They are also very immune suppressant and cause the body to use resources it would normally allocate to maintaining health, tissue elasticity, soft and breathing skin, and preventing cross-linking and hardening of the arteries.

But the greatest damage is the destruction of the cell. Whether it be caused by invading the DNA, breaking the fatty acids in the cell membrane, or destroying the oxygen molecule, the bottom line is the same: premature aging, organ atrophy, auto-immune disorders and cancerous conditions.[23]

Arthritis

Of all the auto-immune disorders, I would specifically like to draw your attention to arthritis. Arthritis is described as a condition where the body's immune system attacks the tissue and membrane between the joints and lubricating fluids.

This is a result of one of the most powerful oxidants known that the body produces: hydroxyl radicals. Hydroxyl radicals are formed when the enzyme xanthine oxidase catalyzes (stimulates) the production of super oxide radicals and hydrogen peroxide (naturally occurring in the body). These free radicals, when mixed with uric acid crystals and sodium hydrogen urate, cause the destruction of the synovial fluids between the joints that provide its lubricating properties.[24] Super oxide radicals are known to break down hyaluronate (the lubricant in joint fluid). The pain and swelling associated with arthritis and gout are the direct result. Rheumatoid arthritis relates to this type of condition where the synovial membranes surrounding the fluid in the joints are attacked. The cartilage and tissues around the joints are destroyed, which the body tries to repair with scar tissue, adding insult to injury by fusing the joints together. Rheumatoid arthritis typically affects the whole body as opposed to osteoarthritis which attacks specific joints, breaking down the cartilage between the joints and the loose ends themselves as they rub together. Lupus (systemic lupus erythematosus) is similar to rheumatoid arthritis in that it is caused by the immune system producing antibodies that attack the body, causing painful, inflamed joints, but which tend not to be crippling.[25]

The anti-oxidants, super oxide dismutase (SOD) and the enzyme catalase protect against this chemical combination happening: super oxide dismutase, by neutralizing the super oxide radicals, and catalase by breaking down hydrogen peroxide.

Dimethyl sulphoxide (DMSO), a solvent used for years to treat animals, is a potent scavenger of hydroxyl free radicals. I typically recommend it for people suffering from arthritic conditions and injuries where scar tissue has had the opportunity to form. It is also excellent for removing scars from surgery or accidents.

DMSO is a powerful solvent that the body converts to a sulphoxide free radical when it destroys a hydroxyl radical. The sulphoxide free radical is then destroyed by the anti-oxidants in the body. As with all of these applications, the key word with DMSO is moderation: less is more.

Most applications are topical, a joint or tissue injury require a razor thin line, applied very sparingly. DMSO is absorbed through the skin, so it is important to have washed the area of application beforehand. You might notice a slight garlic taste; the uptake into the body is very quick and the taste is a residual effect that passes quickly. It is best applied after a shower or bath; but again moderation! Used on a scar, it will diminish it over a period of six to eight months if applied daily over the length of the scar in a razor thin line. Initially the scar may redden, but after a couple of weeks it will begin to disappear.

For joint injuries such as ligament tears in the shoulder, I have recommended a topical application of DMSO taken in conjunction with the homeopathic remedy arnica montana.[26] As the tear heals, the DMSO prevents scar tissue from forming, impeding mobility and putting pressure on the nerves.

DMSO is also very effective in preventing the black and blue marks caused by bruising or crushing injuries. When tissue is damaged by injury, the surrounding blood vessels leak. As the red blood cells hemolyze (break down), iron and copper are released causing free radicals to form as they come in contact with the tissues, which in turn form the black and blue marks. Again use sparingly on clean skin.

Remember for DMSO to be effective it must be taken in conjunction with all the anti-oxidants the body needs.

Other areas of concern regarding free radicals that merit mention

The breasts are particularly vulnerable to free radical damage, since free radicals love to attack polyunsaturated fats (fatty tissue), of which the breasts are primarily composed. Refer to Chapter 4 on colonics where I discussed how breast cancer was traced to the colon – the breasts having provided the ideal dumping ground for toxins carried through the bloodstream and then attacked by its free radicals.

A great strain on anti-oxidant resources is constant exposure to aldehydes, which are cross-linkers, mutagens, carcinogens and acetaldehydes, which are aldehydes made from alcohol in the liver and formed from cigarette smoke and smog pollution.

Many skin disorders are directly related to free radical damage of the cells and the failure of fatty acid cell membrane protection, caused by the sun, radiation and chemicals. Some of these conditions include: psoriasis, eczema and vasculitis.

The sun, essence of all life, also happens to be a killer: through radiation (ultraviolet light exposure). The UVA rays the sun emits penetrate beyond the skin dermis to the cells' first line of defence, melanin, which acts as a filter, absorbing the radiant energy of ultraviolet light. When this defence becomes overwhelmed, the same oxygen radicals that melanin absorbs now attack tissue, damaging lipids, nucleic acids, proteins, proteoglycans and hyaluronic acid. Now it's a free radical free for all. It takes two to three days for new melanin to form; in the meantime free radicals are formed on areas of the skin that have become burned from prolonged exposure, and are caused by airborne bacteria and fungi, drawn to the inflamed area (attracting neutrophils and macrophages which release oxygen radicals through their own respiratory burst). It becomes a 'domino' effect, the result being actinic damage (premature aging of the skin by destruction of the elastic fibre network). This is called cross-linking: an undesirable bond between proteins or nucleic acids (RNA and DNA) wherein the molecules cannot assume the correct shape for proper functioning, thus causing rigidity; a condition also found in hardening of the arteries.

Aging skin is the visual result, the internal one being a carcinogenesis condition or a potentially cancer causing environment. In their 1992 report on free radicals and aging of the skin, Drs Ingrid Emerit and B. Chance[27] found that most Caucasians had already had a certain degree of deterioration of the elastic fibre network characteristic of skin damage by the age of 15 years.

The trick is to keep the cell alive, and the only way to do that is to insulate it through the melanin barrier. We know that it takes 2–3 days after sun exposure for new melanin to form, so the potential for free radical damage during repeated exposure prior to a new melanin barrier forming is extremely high. As melanin absorbs the radiant energy of ultraviolet light, a visible light darkening occurs in its pigments. Melanin also may act as a scavenger of singlet oxygen molecules.

About ten years ago this whole subject of sun exposure began to fascinate me. Living in Southern California and enjoying sunbathing, I decided that there had to be a way to keep the cell alive during exposure to the sun. Once I realized some of the principles discussed above – that the ultraviolet UVA rays once penetrating the melanin barrier go on to destroy the cell, turning it into a free radical – I set about developing a way to bolster the protection available to the cell.

The formula, after a lot of trial and error, finally included anti-oxidants taken as part of a daily regimen and additional ingredients taken a couple of hours before exposure to the sun. While the formula is made up of ingredients taken internally, it does not preclude using a sunscreen of 25 or more.

The result is the desired effect, to tan without burning or free radical damage caused cross-linking (apparent in that criss-cross weaving of lines that appears when you pinch skin together, or obvious on badly damaged skin).

Apart from myself, I tested the formula on many different skin types. I was particularly satisfied with the results on extremely sun sensitive fair skinned individuals. Not only could they tolerate the sun, but did so without the redness or burning that typically occurred after a very brief exposure. These individuals because of pigmentation tend to have very little natural protection.

Maintenance of free radical defences

I am going to list later substances that I personally consider to be excellent formulas; but rather than just listing individual ingredients, I will give a brief description of the ingredients and their properties.

DMAE – H3 (liquid drops)

DMAE[28] (dimethylaminoethanol), the salt and esters of PABA (para-amino benzoic acid) in a concentrated solution, while not an anti-oxidant itself, acts as a scavenger of free radicals, which it then converts so that they can be destroyed by other anti-oxidants. It increases the acetylcholine level in the brain and body, and can dissolve lipofuscin (liver age spots). Acetylcholine releases the hormone vasopressin, a memory learning chemical that regulates motor function, the nervous system sensory response, fluid levels in mucous membranes, urine volume, and gives us drive.

It includes PABA,[29] a B-vitamin, an anti-oxidant, and membrane stabilizer and helps protect red blood cells from bursting (hemolysis), and lysosomal membranes (all) from rupturing and releasing tissue destroying (lysosomal) enzymes. PABA blocks the ultraviolet photons, providing an additional line of defence to melanin in protecting the cell from being blasted by these concentrated particles of light.

Free Radical Quenchers

Beta carotene is one of more than 500 carotenoids, which are found in fruits and vegetables. Carotenoids function as sources of vitamin A, beta carotene having the highest provitamin A activity. Beta carotene's antioxidant properties help prevent against tissue or DNA damage.[30]

Carotenoids' anti-oxidant effects include protection against cancer, particularly lung cancer. The carotenoid lycopene, found abundantly in tomatoes and watermelons, provides anti-oxidant protection against cardiovascular disease.

The same protection carotenoids provide plants from damaging sunlight is provided in the body, preventing photosynthesized oxidation by quenching singlet oxygen. Carotenoids' immune enhancing functions include lymphocyte proliferation, T-helper cells, macrophages[31] and natural killer cell cytotoxicity. There is evidence that carotenoids increase bacterial resistance.

Beta carotene and other carotenoids provide vitamin A on demand to the body, without the toxicity that an oversupply of vitamin A can have.

Glutathione[32] is an important substrate (constituent) for enzymatic anti-oxidant functions, capable of non-enzymatic radical scavenging. It plays a major role in the detoxification of free radicals and toxic oxygen radicals especially in the liver, kidneys, lung, intestines and intracellular oxidants.[33]

Methionine[34] is an essential amino acid (refer to Chapter 6 on amino acids) which acts as a catalyst with other anti-oxidants to detoxify harmful agents, neutralize allergic chemical reactions, and quenche free radical lipid peroxidation. The body converts methionine into homocysteine (an oxidant) then with vitamin B6[35] into anti-oxidant cystathione, so B6 must be a constituent.

N, N-Dimethyglycine (DMG) blocks radiation damage resulting from ultraviolet light.

L-cysteine[36] detoxifies harmful toxins, protects and preserves cells. An anti-oxidant of aldehydes, that cause cross-linking damage from alcohol, smoke, smog, and peroxidized fats.

Ascorbyl palmitate is a lipid soluble vitamin C (fat soluble) and a powerful anti-oxidant synergist.

Alpha tocopherol acetate is a very stable vitamin E ester, in powder form. An important anti-oxidant in protecting against free radical damage and in reversing its effects.

Zinc picolinate[37] is a highly bio-available zinc. Picolinic acid is a zinc binding ligand, which occurs naturally in human breast milk. Zinc is a membrane stabilizer, constituent of the enzyme super oxide dismutase (SOD) preventing cellular damage from super oxide radicals. Always take supplemental zinc with copper using a 30 to 1 ratio.

Selenium[38] (NASE) is an important anti-oxidant mineral, part of the enzyme glutathione peroxidase, which protects the body from peroxides. Works with other anti-oxidants, vitamin E and cysteine.

Ubiquinone[39] (CoQ[10]) is an anti-oxidant, which protects against lipid peroxidation by removing excess molecules of oxygen, and neutralizing free radical oxygen renegades.

Lipoic acid[40] (or thioctic acid) is an anti-oxidant, which interacts with reactive oxygen species such as super oxide anion and hydroxide preventing lipid peroxidation. It is also anti-viral; recent research concerns its ability to inhibit human immunodeficiency virus (HIV-1) replication.

Formula for daily free radical defence

The formula, which is also a daily maintenance regimen for free radical defence, is as follows:

Anti-mutagens	x 2
Co-enzyme B-complex	x 2
Vitamin C – Ester and Quericitin	x 2(1,000 mg)
Viricidin – Lauricidin ©	x 2
OxyCaps (Sodium Chlorite/Sodium Carbonate)	
Amino acids complex (18 aminos)	x 3
Free Radical Quenchers	x 2
DMAE (full stopper, mixed in juice)	1 ml

Taken with a non-acid (papaya) juice (8 ounces) on an empty stomach, upon rising (morning) with no food or beverage for 45–60 minutes.

This is a complete free radical defence formula, not only from radiation damage due to ultraviolet light but also from environmental pollutants such as smog, smoke, auto-exhaust, and chemical additives. It is also an internal defence against auto-immune conditions caused by toxins in the body. This line of defence extends to the various free radical categories caused also by dietary induced chemical reactions, such as lipid peroxidation (fats), super oxide radicals, and hydroxyl radicals.

By having the resources available to do battle with the millions of free radicals we are bombarded with daily, we keep our cells alive. We stop the antigens and mutagens that would attack our DNA and RNA, aging our bodies much faster than our biological clock.

As I have mentioned earlier, this has become a major part of my own personal research; aging and why we have to age? If every cell in our body is replaced over a seven year cycle (other than our teeth), then why during that cycle do our organs, tissue, bones, etc. have to atrophy and age? A significant part of my discovery in this area is that we do not have to age. Free radical damage breaks down our growth and rebuilding abilities as the body devotes all of its resources to fighting the daily bombardment. Most people's immune systems are so overloaded, dealing with conditions (acute or chronic) which, compounded with environmental pollutants and devitalized diets, have left them with no ability to mount an offensive, or to rebuild or reverse atrophied conditions, because the immune system is always disadvantaged.

I remember reading a study done in 1970 on GIs who were killed in Vietnam, whose average age was 20. The autopsy results showed that their major organs were twice their physical age. This was attributed to being the first generation raised on a supermarket diet. Not only that, but they were also the first generation raised on devitalized processed food, full of free radical forming additives.

You now have the tools to change that situation,
to reprogram your body for help, and
to halt the aging process.

12

Blood Chemistry[41]

The body, as I have already mentioned, is like a chemistry laboratory; and now you get to play chief technician. To do this you need to have a blood test, either by a registered clinic (they can usually mail or fax your results within two or three days) or your health care practitioner, who is obliged to provide you with a copy of your results upon request.

Your blood test results will come in the form of what is known as a 24 panel chemical screen and a CBC (or complete blood count). The 24 chemical screen details all the constituents of blood plasma – the pinkish/red fluid, 95% water, which contains nutrients, proteins, waste products and hormones in a saline solution similar to sea water.

The nutrients, which include amino acids, fats, sugars, vitamins, and minerals, are either transported from the intestinal tract or released from the liver. Their levels indicate the amount of fuel available to the body in the following way.

Amino acids form three quarters of the dry weight of most body cells. They are the building blocks in the biochemical structure of enzymes, hormones, antibodies, and nutrient carriers. They are divided into two categories: essential – those the body must ingest, and non-essential – those the body produces. (Refer to Chapter 6 on amino acids.)

Fats provide the cells (mitochondria – part of the cell that converts fats to energy) with over 90% of their source of energy. The mitochondrion is the organelle responsible for releasing energy from fats. These fatty acids break down into two categories: saturated – fats that contain no carbon to carbon double bonds and highly saturated with hydrogen atoms which become rancid and toxic when excessively heated and ingested causing auto-oxidation; and polyunsaturated – fats that contain two or more double bonds between some of their carbon atoms, lacking hydrogen concentration (very susceptible to auto-oxidation when heated, becoming carcinogenic, immune suppressive, cross-linked and peroxidized).

Sugars are another source of cellular fuel, including glucose or blood sugar. Regulated by insulin (lowers) and glucagon (raises) from pancreas, thyroid hormone, liver enzymes and adrenal hormones. The liver converts carbohydrates (monosaccharides, disaccharides, polysaccharides), lactic acid, proteins and fats into glucose.

Vitamins are essential nutrients for the body's function. Divided into two categories: fat soluble vitamins – A,D,E and K which are absorbed with fats from the intestine and stored mainly in the liver to be used as required; and water soluble vitamins – C, all the B vitamins, which the body uses immediately and is unable to store (any superfluous to use is indicated by a dark or yellow coloured urine after ingestion).

Minerals are essential to the body's functions and include potassium, calcium, sodium, magnesium, phosphorus and trace elements of iron, zinc, and copper.

Waste products are produced as the byproduct of normal metabolism. They show up in the blood in the following ways: BUN (blood urea nitrogen), the nitrogen part of urea, an end product of protein breakdown. Urea is formed in the liver and excreted by the kidneys. Uric acid is the end product of purine metabolism from cell nucleic acids. Carbon dioxide is a waste product of energy production from carbohydrates and fats which is eliminated through the respiratory exchange of carbon dioxide in the lungs. Biliruben is the haemoglobin from dead red blood cells. It is transported to the liver, and converted to bile.

Proteins are of two principal types: fibrous and globular. Fibrous proteins make up many of the body's tissues, like collagen, the major structural molecule of the body. Collagen comprises 30% of total body protein and is a principal constituent of connective tissue, muscle, skin, hair, cartilage and the vascular system. Globular proteins are the soluble proteins that the liver forms to carry enzymes, hormones, lipids, haemoglobin and is the gamma portion of the immune system, containing antibodies.

Hormones are produced by the endocrine system, which is made up of adrenals, pancreas, parathyroid glands, pituitary gland, thyroid, testes, and ovaries. The kidneys, intestines and brain also produce certain hormones. Hormones produced by the endocrine system regulate body functions such as metabolism, growth, sexual development, and the immune response to stress or illness. They act as chemical messengers, using the bloodstream as a highway.

Blood chemistry results

To return to your blood test. The results will provide you with a snap shot of your blood chemistry at the time the sample was taken. It will reflect all the elements, enzymes, and chemicals, and their correlation to laboratory values, reflecting a mean or range from a reference population. This range is established by a computation of results from thousands of blood tests.

Typically you want to be somewhere in the middle of the range, which is the mean. For example, if the range for potassium is 3.4–5.2 mEq/L, the mean would be 4.3 mEq/L. A deviation higher or lower may represent overload or deficiency, and the extent depending on how far the deviation is from the mean. I have found that elevated and deficient levels usually correlate, and that you can establish a pattern and target for problem areas. The following will enable you to read your own blood test results.

The reference ranges or laboratory values can vary from laboratory to laboratory. Most laboratories establish these values by using a cross-section of the thousands of blood samples they analyze. Since the samples include both the healthiest along with the most unhealthy, they subtract a percentage from the top and the bottom to establish normal ranges.

The laboratory ranges may vary slightly, so you may want to determine how close you are to the mean. The mean is the centre of the range and considered the number for optimum health. As you get further from the mean towards the low or high end of the range, you need to determine where the deficiency or overload is coming from. The conditions listed are some of the typical indications.

Because you are in the range of values does not mean everything is OK; laboratories only flag those values that are out of range. I have had many people hand me their blood work having been told that everything was fine. A more careful scrutiny revealed chronic or even acute conditions that went untreated because the values were just over or under the range. Obviously if you are out of the range on either end, this is much more of a flashing red light and easier to identify problem areas. But pay attention to how close you are to the mean; also look at the complete picture, not just one or two readings and try to establish a pattern. Think of your blood work as a puzzle; all the pieces are there and they all fit together to form a picture of a healthy you.

The *Système International* (SI) is the metric-based laboratory data reporting system used in Europe and Canada. Even though some countries use the units per litre U/L (USA) system for measuring enzymatic activity, depending where you are, you may find the values on your results in either U/L or SI or a combination of both. When using the SI system, determine the middle of the range to establish the mean.

Fasting Glucose

Glucose is the primary source of energy (blood sugar) for cells. Regulated by insulin and glucagon from the pancreas, thyroid hormone, liver enzymes, and adrenal hormones. The liver converts lactic acid, proteins, and fats into glucose.
Range: 65–115 mg/dL   (SI:3.89–5.83 nmol/L)
Mean: 87.5 mg/dL

Low end of range may indicate excess insulin, liver disease, poor absorption, hypothyroidism, or alcoholism. Elevated levels indicate stress, diabetes, liver damage, hyperthyroidism, pancreatitis, or use of oral contraceptives.

BUN

Blood urea nitrogen (BUN) is the end product of nucleic acid (DNA and RNA), caused by amino acids in metabolism by the cells. Nitrogen is a byproduct that becomes part of the urea formed in the liver. The liver passes it on to the kidneys to be excreted.
Range: 8–23 mg/dL   (SI:1.8–7.1 mmol/L)
Mean: 15.5 mg/dL

Low end of range may indicate poor protein uptake, poor nutrient assimilation, liver damage, pancreas or adrenal atrophy or pregnancy. Elevated levels indicate excessive protein intake, kidney damage, poor hydration (fluid intake), liver or thyroid damage, intestinal haemor-rhaging, or presence of pharmaceutical drugs (certain types).

Creatinine

Creatinine is a byproduct of muscle metabolism. The level reflects muscle metabolism: when the body is starved or protein digestion impaired, muscles break down to supply amino acids.
Range: 0.7–1.4 mg/dL   (SI: 97 μmol/L)
Mean: 1.1 mg/dL

Low end of range indicates starvation, impaired protein digestion, liver disease, kidney damage or pregnancy. Elevated levels can indicate kidney damage or disease since creatinine is eliminated by the kidneys. Muscle degeneration or drugs that impair kidneys may also be indicated.

BUN/Creatine Ratio

If the level is elevated, then too much BUN is being formed. A low level can indicate that creatine is not being eliminated by the kidneys. This blood marker is an important indicator of kidney and liver function, and protein metabolism.
Range: 6–20
Mean: 10

Sodium

Sodium plays a vital role in not only the blood but also in many body functions. In the blood it is a principal electrolyte (positively charged cation), responsible for charging the body's electrical system. Sodium serves to regulate blood pressure, and blood pH, produce digestive

fluids, stabilize acid balance, and facilitate nerve function. It also controls the thickness of the blood, maintains homeo-static balance of cells, and muscle function. Its level is regulated by the kidneys and adrenal glands.
Range: 135–148 mEq/L   (SI:136–147 mmol/L)
Mean: 141.5 mEq/L

Low end of range can indicate low blood sugar, weakness, dehydration, lethargy and heart palpitation. It may also indicate kidney malfunction and acidic condition.

Elevated levels indicate hypertension, anaemia, kidney and liver disease. Also, because it needs to balanced with potassium, excessive sodium can lead to a potassium deficiency, and then to heart disease.

Potassium

The alter-ego of sodium, another principal (intracellular) electrolyte carrying a positive charge (cation). It maintains a healthy nervous system and is critical to heart function. It works in conjunction with sodium to regulate water balance, especially on a cellular level. It is a catalyst for many important chemical reactions within the cells and the transfer of nutrients into the cells. Potassium contributes to maintaining blood pressure and for electrical conduction in the nerves and muscles. It is needed for hormonal secretion.
Range: 3.4–5.3 mEq/L   (SI:3.5–5 mmol/L)
Mean: 4.3 mEq/L

Low end of range may indicate loss due to kidney disorders, diarrhoea, or use of diuretics and laxatives. It may also indicate stress, poor nutrition, excess insulin, rapid heart beat, and nervous system malfunction. Elevated levels indicate diabetes, trauma, kidney disease, myocardial infarction, slow heart beat, and respiratory disease.

Chloride

This is another electrolyte, only negatively charged (anion), which serves to maintain the acid and alkaline levels. It transports fluid exchange across cell membranes and helps regulate blood pressure, blood volume, and the osmotic pressure of blood. It is also needed for production of hydrochloride acid in the stomach.
Range: 95–109 mEq/L   (SI:97 – 107 mmol/L)
Mean: 102 mEq/L

Low end of range may indicate low sodium intake, fluid retention, kidney disease, poor nutrition, and diarrhoea. Symptoms may be indigestion, intestinal gas, dry skin, tendency to hyperventilate, and experiencing heat exhaustion. Elevated levels will reflect acidosis, renal failure, severe dehydration, and hyperventilation.

Carbon Dioxide

Carbon Dioxide (CO_2) is exchanged in the lungs during respiration for oxygen. CO_2 is the byproduct of glucose picked up by red blood cells and carried via the heart to the lungs. It is one of the end products of nutrient metabolism in the cells.

Range: 20–32 mEq/L   (SI:20–29 mmol/L)
Mean: 25.5 mEq/L

Low CO_2 levels may be due to poor nutrition (starvation), uraemia (kidney malfunction), respiratory alkalosis (decrease in oxygen carrying capacity of blood), or metabolic acidosis (hyperventilation) due to diabetic acidosis, aspirin ingestion or alcoholism. It also may indicate central nervous system disease and liver malfunction. Elevated levels can be a result of severe vomiting, or not getting enough oxygen or volume of air to expel CO_2. Drugs such as cortisone or diuretics will increase its levels.

Calcium

Calcium is the principal constituent of strong bones and teeth, which both act as repositories to service the body's needs. Calcium maintains a regular heartbeat and regulates nerve impulses. It is also needed for muscle growth and contraction. Calcium is essential in blood clotting (coagulation), helps regulate cell membrane permeability and lowers blood pressure. It is very dependent on hormonal activity (thyroid gland, parathyroid glands, adrenal steroids, vitamin D), metabolic changes, acid/alkaline ratio, and phosphorous (requires the amino acid lysine for absorption). Calcium provides energy and participates in the protein structuring of RNA/DNA.

Range: 8.5–10.5 mg/dL   (SI:2.05–2.54 mmol/L)
Mean: 9.5 mg/dL

Low levels of calcium can be due to devitalized diet, kidney dysfunction, hormone imbalance, hypoparathyroidism, or vitamin D deficiency. Indicators may be muscle cramps, nervousness, heart palpitations, eczema, hypertension, higher cholesterol levels, rheumatoid arthritis, tooth decay, insomnia, and numbness in limbs.

Elevated levels are indicative of hyperparathyroidism, hyperthyroidism, bone tumours, or elevated vitamin D levels. Constant use of antacids can contribute to elevated levels due to the active ingredient calcium carbonate, which neutralizes stomach acid needed for proper metabolism. Higher levels can lead to deficiency of zinc, which, like calcium, is another extremely important mineral in the body's chemistry.

Phosphorus

With calcium it is a constituent of and catalyst to the formation of bone, teeth and cells. It is abundant in cells and tissue, and it is needed to form the energy bonds for carbohydrate metabolism. Forms part of cell membrane (phospholipids) used to convert vitamins and nutrients into fuel (energy).

Range: 2.5–4.5 mg/dL   (SI:0.81–1.45 mmol/L)
Mean: 3.5 mg/dL

Low levels can indicate a hyperacidic condition, hyperparathyroidism, vitamin D deficiency or liver disease. Contributors may be a devitalized diet or alcoholism. Pregnancy and lactation may also produce a low reading. Elevated levels can indicate kidney disease, hypothyroidism, diabetes, liver disease or an alkaline digestive tract. Excessive vitamin D intake, as in junk food diets, can be contributors.

Uric acid

A byproduct of protein metabolism, uric acid is found in the blood and eliminated through the kidneys as urine.

Range: 3.7–7.6 mg/dL   (SI:202–416 μmol/L)
Mean: Male – 5.65 mg/dL
        Female – 4.35 mg/dL

Low levels indicate a low protein diet, kidney disease, liver atrophy or poor absorption of nutrients from the gastrointestinal tract. A contributor can be an acid kidney eliminating too quickly.

Elevated levels are associated with kidney disease, infections, gout, or auto-immune disorders. Contributors can be an excess of alcohol or protein or an alkaline kidney eliminating poorly.

Albumin

When all the amino acids (essential and non-essential) have assembled in the liver, protein is manufactured. Albumin is a protein produced by the liver and is correlated to the protein adequacy of the diet. It controls nutrient transport (fatty acids, vitamins, minerals, hormones, and biliruben), and fluid retention (oedema), because it maintains osmotic pressure and waste removal.

Range: 3.5–5 g/dL   (SI:35–50 g/L)
Mean: 4.25 g/dL

Low levels indicate inadequate protein uptake (deficient diet), liver disease, gastric disorders, poor blood viscosity, fever, infection (inflammation of kidneys, glomerulonephritis) or haemorrhage. Pregnancy and lactation will also be reflected in lower levels. Elevated levels can represent dehydration, shock, localized or widespread malignant tumours of the bone marrow or liver disease.

Total Protein

By adding the albumin and globulin in the blood, you arrive at the total protein produced by the liver.
Range: 6.3–8.3 g/dL
Mean: 6.85 g/dL

Globulin

Also formed in the liver, globulin carries some hormones, lipids, and metals. Gamma-globulin refers to antibodies produced by the immune system. A gamma-globulin breakdown (into types A, G, M and E) is necessary for diagnosis of certain infections and allergies.
Range: 2.0–5.0 g/dL
Mean: 2.8 g/dL
    Lower levels may indicate immune deficiency, impaired protein digestion or malnutrition. It can also represent anaemia, liver or kidney disease. Elevated readings will denote chronic infections, cirrhotic liver condition, rheumatoid arthritis, myeloma, and lupus.

Albumin / Globulin Ratio

This reading will be out of range due to conditions affecting the globulin level.
Range: 1.1–2.5
Mean: 1.7

Cholesterol

Cholesterol is one of the most important anti-oxidants made by the body. It protects cell membranes and is needed for membrane synthesis and repair. The liver produces most of the cholesterol in the blood, the rest is absorbed from dietary factors. Cholesterol helps form the hormones of the adrenal cortex, without which all sorts of immune deficient, auto-immune disorders would result. A complex interaction exists between adrenal hormones and immune function.
Range: 121–304 mg/dL   (SI:3.12–7.86 mmol/L)
Mean: 200 mg/dL
    Lower level readings (below 150) indicate an impaired immune system or adrenal inadequacy. Levels lower than 130 are indicative of cancer activity. Because of the effect of lowered hormones produced by the adrenal cortex, the immune system is debilitated and auto-immune

disorders, ranging from arthritis to all types of opportunistic infections, may develop. The heart can also be affected, developing into (fatal) cardiac arrhythmia.

Elevated levels will be reflected in the presence of heart disease, arteriosclerosis, liver disease, diabetes, hypothyroidism or genetic (inherited) weakness. High cholesterol will also indicate immune deficiency.

Low Density Lipoproteins (fat-protein molecules) (LDL)

These carry cholesterol to the tissues. When deposited in the lining of your arteries, white blood cells called phagocytes attach to the cholesterol and eat it. In the process the phagocytes produce a number of oxygen-related free radicals causing the cholesterol to become oxidized. The oxidized cholesterol is now a mutagen and plaque causing agent. The formation of plaque prevents the synthesis of the anti-clotting factor, prostacyclin (PG1) in the arterial walls. Prostacyclin is now unavailable to prevent red blood cells from attaching to the plaque and arterial walls. As the red blood cells leak iron and copper, more free radical oxidation hastens the process of plaque formation. LDL can be especially carcinogenic since it can carry into the bloodstream the toxic tar residue inhaled into the lungs from auto-exhausts, cigarette smoke, smog, etc.

High Density Lipoproteins (fat-protein molecules) (HDL)

These are called the good cholesterol, or blood lipid fractions that remove cholesterol from the arteries and tissues. This is the anti-oxidant cholesterol which responds to LDL or serum cholesterol levels based on the amount of anti-oxidants at its disposal. Also controls blood clotting whereby thromboxane, which forms platelet clusters, is prevented from abnormal clotting by prostacyclin. We know that elevated LDL levels interfere with prostacyclin.

The secret to controlling or reducing LDL and maintaining HDL at a 2 to 1 ratio with LDL is anti-oxidants, particularly those that include vitamins A, E, C, B1, B5, B6, and the amino acids, glutathione, cysteine, and methionine, the minerals zinc, selenium, and anti-mutagens. Chromium, though not an anti-oxidant, has properties similar to anti-oxidants in its ability to protect the cells (avoid chromium chloride). This provides for a strong immune system that works in conjunction with the HDL destroying antigens and mutagens before they can do damage and overwhelm the immune system. Most importantly, avoid peroxidized fats and oils (foods and oils that have been exposed to oxygen and gone rancid), especially flesh foods, cooked oils, grains etc.

Triglycerides

Free floating fatty acids (fat soluble vitamins and acids) are absorbed into the bloodstream via the small intestine, or converted from glucose. Stored in the mitochondria (energy producing organelles) of the liver, fatty acids are oxidized to produce ATP (adenosine) triphosphate, the cells' universal energy molecule. The liver produces proteins for carrying the triglyceride energy molecule to the heart and kidneys as fuel.

Range: 40–160 mg/dL   (SI:0.45–1.81 mmol/L)
Mean: 90 mg/dL

Low level readings may indicate poor protein synthesis or impaired fatty acid absorption by the liver (ability to store). Other indicators may be hypoglycaemia, and stress related disorders. Protein impaired synthesis can affect connective tissue (collagen formation), muscle tissue and blood vessels.

Elevated levels reflect fatty acid accumulation,[42] which may have toxic effects on cell function and may result in an intracellular energy deficit. Other indicators may be diabetes, kidney disease, liver disease, pancreatitis, biliary (bile duct) blockage, alcoholism, and heart conditions (arrhythmia, myopathy).

In low readings, supplement with B vitamins, especially B6 (pyridoxine hydrochloride), B3 (niacin), and B5 (pantothenic acid). These should be taken in conjunction with the fatty acids linoleic acid, gamma-linolenic acid, and alpha-linolenic acid. Zinc is needed also as a catalyst for fatty acid utilization.

Higher levels can be effectively reduced using L-carnitine, chromium piconolate, or B3 (niacin). L-carnitine and niacin increase the metabolism of fat into fuel. Chromium piconolate improves glucose tolerance by reducing insulin requirements, and stimulates lipid metabolism to reduce total cholesterol, LDL, and triglycerides, and increase HDL cholesterol. These should be taken also in conjunction with the protocol for low levels, B-complex, omega 6 series (linoleic, gamma, alpha), and zinc.

Total Biliruben

This is the waste product from dead red blood cells and their haemoglobin. It reflects the liver's eliminative function, since biliruben is deposited into the liver to be converted into bile and eliminated into the intestines via the bile duct.

Range: 0.1–1.2 mg/dL   (SI:3.4–17.1 µmol/L)
Mean: 0.65 mg/dL

Low level readings indicate the liver or spleen may be malfunctioning or that iron deficient anaemia is producing insufficient red blood cells.

If elevated, the indicators may be viral hepatitis, liver disease, bile duct obstruction or haemolytic anaemia. Any of these will cause red blood cells to be rapidly destroyed either because of their abnormal shape and function or because the liver cannot process the amount being produced.

With lower levels, take homeopathic ferrum phosphoricum sublingually (under the tongue) to offset iron deficient anaemia (this gets it right into the blood stream, as opposed to ingesting, where iron turns to a chloride in the stomach). Try to avoid barbiturates and aspirin, which lower biliruben readings.

Elevated levels, depending on the cause, can be helped with silymarin, excellent for rebuilding the liver and preventing further damage from conditions contributing to the problem. Anti-inflammatories can be used such as vitamin C with bioflavanoids, ginger root, tumeric, and alpha omega fatty acids.

Taking anti-oxidants will also help prevent a further breakdown of red blood cell membranes, and help the immune system deal with the problem.

Direct Biliruben

This indicates the liver's ability to convert haemoglobin into water-soluble substances that can be eliminated through the kidneys.
Range: 0.0–0.3 mg/dL   (SI:<3.4 µmol/L)
Mean: 0.2 mg/dL

Low levels indicate fatigue, adrenal gland exhaustion or viral infection. Elevated levels can represent liver disease, mononucleosis (glandular fever) or gall stones. Refer to protocols for total biliruben.

Alkaline Phosphatase

This is an enzyme found primarily in the liver, but also prevalent in bone and intestinal mucosa. Higher levels are usually caused by cell damage, repair or rapid growth. Since alkaline phosphatase regulates mineral transport in and out of the bones, injury to the bones will reflect higher levels.
Range: 39–118 IU/L
Children: 50–400 IU/L
Mean: 75 IU/L

Low levels can reflect adrenal exhaustion, anaemia or hypothyroidism. Zinc and folic acid deficiencies can also contribute, because zinc is an enzymatic co-factor required for alkaline phosphatase synthesis. Protein deficiency, magnesium, vitamin C, and B12 deficiencies will also produce lower levels.

Elevated levels are an indicator of liver disease, bone disease and mononucleosis. Pharmaceutical drugs will also raise levels and toxic deposits in the liver. Children will show elevated levels due to bone growth.

LDH

Lactic dehydrogenase is an enzyme found in most organs, kidneys, liver, brain, lungs, and especially the heart. It is also found on muscles and blood serum.

Range: 94–250 IU/L
Mean: 182.5 IU/L

Low levels can be caused by nutrient deficiency (malnutrition), adrenal exhaustion, hypoglycaemia or organ and muscle atrophy. Elevated readings are to be found in heart attack victims (myocardial infarction), where levels will be their highest up to four days after the attack. Leukemia, anaemia, liver disease, lung embolus (blood clot), pancreatitis, and tissue damage from cancer or injury also reveal elevated readings.

GGT (Gamma Glutamyl Transepeptidase)

This is a liver enzyme. One of the globular protein constituents (enzymes) that promotes chemical reactions in the body.

Range: 9–50 U/L
Mean: 25 U/L

It is low in hypothyroidism (underactive), hypothalamic malfunction (thyroid hormone is needed for proper function of immune system), or magnesium deficiency. Higher levels usually indicate a bile duct obstruction, liver disease, pancreatitis (inflammation) or alcohol related conditions. Elevated magnesium intake will also give a higher reading.

SGOT (AST) (Serum Glutamic Oxaloacetic Transaminase)

This is also a glandular liver enzyme, found in the heart, liver, kidneys, pancreas, and muscles. In the liver it is an enzyme used to detoxify and neutralize chemicals and pollutants. Remember that one-third of the liver's weight is made up of kuppfer cells, which are phagocytic cells (responsible for isolating and killing invading bacteria) which neutralize toxins and bacteria before they can do damage.

Range: 10–40 U/L
Mean: 25.5 U/L

Low levels, below 10 U/L, usually indicate a B-vitamin deficiency or pregnancy. Elevated levels are much more complex: levels above 40 U/L show up in liver related disorders, i.e. inflammation of the liver (hepatitis), viral, bacterial, fungal or parasitic infections. Also kidney and muscle damage or infection and mononucleosis can elevate levels. SGOT levels are used to monitor heart attack victims since levels increase up to 20 times over the normal in the 24 hour period after the heart attack.

Selenium deficiency is associated with elevated levels, and it is important to note that four atoms of selenium are part of every molecule of the anti-oxidant (anti-aging) enzyme glutathione peroxidase.

SGPT (ALT) (Serum Glutamic Pyruvic Transaminase)

Also a globular liver enzyme, to a lesser extent found in heart muscle and other tissues.
Range: 10–40 U/L
Mean: 18.5 U/L

Lower levels below 10 U/L indicate poorly oxygenated tissues. Elevated levels above 40 U/L are indicative of the same conditions of SGOT associated levels, i.e. liver inflammation and disorders due to viral, bacterial, fungal or parasitic infections.

For SGOT and SGPT lowering elevated levels of both requires detoxifying and rebuilding liver function. Suggestions for tackling both are:
Detoxifying = Antioxidants
  – Vitamins A, C, E, B-complex.
  – Selenium, zinc, lipoic acid.
  – Choline, methionine, L-cysteine.
Rebuilding and Healing
  – Silymarin (milk thistle), turmeric, licorice root.
  – Ginger, beet juice/powder, chlorella, garlic.

Iron

Iron is vital for the productions of a number of proteins, haemoglobin, myoglobun, and cytochrome. Most of the iron required by the body is used in bone marrow to make haemoglobin (in red blood cells).

Haemoglobin carries oxygen from the lungs to the billion cells and tissues where it is exchanged for carbon dioxide. An adult will contain 3–4 grams of iron, half of which will be found in the haemoglobin, up to a gram stored in the liver, and the rest at various sites throughout the body.
Range: 50–170 µg/dL   (SI:8.95–30.43 µmol/L)
Mean: 87.5 µg/dL

Lower levels or deficiency, below 55 µg/dL, causes oxygen deprivation to the body's cells. Low levels also create immune suppressant conditions, i.e. atrophy of lymphoid tissues,[43] decreasing both T-cell lymphocytes[44] which form antibodies to fight antigens and disease. They also impair neutrophils (phagocytes) responsible for isolating and killing bacteria causing infection. Other conditions include anaemia, low hydrochloric acid, aging, liver disease, and excessive menstrual flow. Elevated levels, above 120 µug/dL, are even more immune suppressant than too little iron, reducing neutrophils necessary for isolating and killing circulating bacteria, viruses or antigens. High levels of inorganic iron destroys vitamin E, which protects the cell membrane from free radical damage. Without this protection the red blood cells haemolyze (burst) releasing iron which is oxidized, creating more free radicals that feed on healthy cells. Pathogens and cancer cells feed on iron. Auto-immune conditions such as rheumatoid arthritis are promoted by this (free radical) reactive process to excessive inorganic iron levels.

Too much iron is as bad as too little. Both are extremely immune suppressant. The key is to try to reduce inorganic iron and replace it with organic iron. Iron that has been added to processed foods is inorganic, so you need to eat a lot of anti-oxidants to protect the cells, especially vitamin E. Refering back to the chapter on cell salts (Chapter 8) you will remember that ferrum phosphoricum is the best way to get supplement organic iron, since 50% is stored in the bloodstream. Another way is to give blood. This will reduce levels, which you can then monitor with diet and by giving blood periodically until levels stabilize.

TIBC (Total Iron Binding Capacity)

This reading is an important one since it relates to access and binding availability of iron storage sites in the blood stream.
Range: 250–450 µg/dL)   (SI:44.75–80.55 µmol/L)
Mean: 350 µg/dL

Lower levels indicate anaemia of infection and chronic disease, cirrhosis of liver, haemochromatosis (where iron pigments are deposited in tissues throughout the body), nephrosis (degeneration of the kidneys).

Elevated levels indicate iron deficiency, anaemia, acute or chronic blood loss, hepatitis, or the use of oral contraceptives.

Iron / TIBC ratio

This level indicates the percentage of iron binding sites saturated with iron.
Range: 20–50%

Lower levels below 15% indicate iron deficiency anaemia, and that there are many iron binding sites available. Elevated levels are representative of haemochromatosis, where there are skin colour changes, cirrhosis of the liver and diabetes. All available binding sites are full.

Blood

Our vascular freeway system carries nutrients from the intestines through the liver, then out to the cells. From the cells it exchanges nutrients for waste products, carrying them back to the liver for detoxification and elimination. It takes oxygen and glucose to the cells and exchanges it for carbon dioxide, which it carries back to the lungs. The blood is composed of two major parts, plasma, which contains all of the nutrients, waste products and proteins discussed so far and the blood cells, which make up 50% of the blood's volume. Red blood cells are manufactured by the bone marrow, through divisions from a single type of cell called a stem cell. These are cells which remain in an immature state of development until they are needed to replace cells that have died. The ends of the long bones, and especially the ribs and sternum, are the source of red blood cell production.

White blood cells are manufactured by the lymphatic tissue, specifically the lymphatic glands, and enter the blood stream through the lymph system. Bone marrow contributes to the production of the eosinophil cells in white blood cells. So you have Red blood cells (erythrocytes) for oxygen transport, White blood cells (leucocytes) for fighting infection, and Platelets (thrombocytes) for blood clotting.

Red Blood Cells (RBC)

RBCs are doughnut-shaped, with between 4.1–6.1 million per cubic millimetre (mean 4.8 million per cubic millimetre) of blood. They contain the pigment and protein haemoglobin. The red blood cells carry oxygen to the tissues and carbon dioxide back to the lungs:
Range: 4.18–5.48 m/µl (SI:4.18–5.48 10^{12}/L
Mean: 4.80 m/µl

Low readings, below 4.1 million per cubic millimetre are usually associated with anaemia, poor nutrition absorption or a nutrient deficient diet. (Iron, and vitamins B12 and B6 are all needed to make RBCs.)

Elevated levels above 6.1 million per cubic millimetre indicate a blood toxicity. For example, nitrates from food bind with haemoglobin to produce methaemogubun, which prevents oxygen from being transported. This causes the bone marrow to accelerate manufacture of RBCs to offset oxygen deprivation. Liver or spleen malfunction (polycythaemia – a disease associated with enlarged spleen), and bone marrow disease are indicative of elevated levels. Deficiencies of vitamins B12, and B6, folic acid or too much iron (which creates separate immune system problems) will also increase levels.

White Blood Cells (WBC)

White blood cells (leucocytes) make up 1% of our blood, averaging 7 thousand per cubic millimetre of blood, compared to 5 million red cells. The white blood cells are those associated with the immune system and come in a number of shapes and sizes. They have fascinating chameleon capabilities, constantly changing their form, and have stealth capabilities, allowing them to exit blood vessel walls into the extravascular spaces to protect the body against viruses, bacteria, fungi, parasites or any infection. They come in three categories, which then divide up again into individual groups, each with a specific purpose. These individual varieties are identified in a white blood count panel.

The three types are:

Granulocytes (or polymorphonuclear leukocytes)
 – Neutrophils (or phagocytes)
 – Basophils
 – Eosinophils
Monocytes (type of phagocyte)
Lymphocytes
 – B-type lymphocytes
 – T-type lymphocytes

The white blood cell count is a measure of the disease fighting availability of the blood.

Range: 3.8–10.8 K/μL (SI:3.8–10.8, 10^9/L)
Mean: 7.15 K/μL

Levels below 4.8 suggest an immune system crisis: disease or infection has gained a foothold and is overwhelming it. Look at the individual white blood count breakdown to try and isolate the immune deficiency. An elevated WBC count, above 10.8, usually indicates a bacterial infection. Check the differential count of granulocytes.

Haemoglobin (HBC)

The haemoglobin is the pigment in the red blood cells, which is the protein that carries oxygen to the cells and tissues.

Range: 13.5–18.0 g/dL (SI:135–180 g/L)
Mean: 14.8 g/dL

Low levels below 13.5 are usually associated with anaemia due to lack of iron in diet, poor nutrition, or a malabsorption condition. Levels above 18.0 indicate toxic interference (such as nitrates), causing oxygen deprivation and stimulating the liver to produce excessive haemoglobin to compensate. If too much iron is being ingested, the liver and spleen will malfunction, also causing elevated levels.

Haematocrit (HCT)

The haematocrit is a measure of the relative proportion of red blood cells to plasma.
Range: 35–52 %
Mean: 44 %
Lower levels, below 44%, are usually associated with anaemia, by over hydration (too much fluid). An overactive spleen can also bring the percentage down. Elevated levels, above 52%, can be caused by dehydration (too little fluid) or a reduced breakdown of RBCs by the spleen.

Mean Corpuscular Volume (MCV)

The mean corpuscular volume indicates the size of red blood cells.
Range: 81–99 μm^3 (SI:80-100 fL)
Mean: 90 μm^3
Low levels, below 81, are associated with microcytic anaemia, where the RBCs are abnormally small, creating a haemoglobin deficiency and consequently preventing oxygen from getting to the cells. Elevated levels, above 99, usually mean macrocytic anaemia, caused by abnormally large RBCs that the spleen has not destroyed.

Mean Corpuscular Haemoglobin (MCH)

Mean corpuscular haemoglobin gives the average weight of the haemoglobin found in RBCs.
Range: 27–35 pg (SI:27.0–33.7 pg)
Mean: 30 pg
Low levels below 27 are usually associated with light coloured RBCs from an iron deficiency. Elevated levels reflect an increased amount of haemoglobin in the RBCs due to inadequate or poor oxygenation.

Mean Corpuscular Haemoglobin Concentration (MCHC)

The MCHC indicates if the average RBC is anaemic.
Range: 30–36 g/dL (SI:330–370 g/L)
Mean: 33 g/dL
Low levels are associated with hypo-chronic anaemia, an RBC deficiency and a greater haemoglobin deficiency. Elevated levels are associated with hyper-chronic anaemia, where the RBC deficiency is greater than the haemoglobin deficiency.

Platelet (thrombocytes) Count

Formed in the bone marrow daily, hundreds of million platelets (irregularly shaped, colourless, and about one-third the size of RBCs) enter the bloodstream. Platelets contribute to the blood clotting process, providing thrombin to form a clot to stop a bleeding blood vessel or burn. The negative aspect of blood clotting is that when arterial walls have thickened due to atherosclerosis (hardening of the arteries), clots can form an embolus or thrombus with serious consequences.

Range: 150–450 K/μL (SI:150–450 10⁹/L)
Mean: 300 K/μL

Levels below 150 indicate immune system failure. Drug ingestion will also cause low levels, as will vitamin B12 or folic acid deficiencies. Elevated levels are usually associated with dehydration.

Headaches, although not directly related to elevated platelet levels, can be influenced by them. Each platelet is made up of bacteria killers, clotting factors, and small bundles of adrenaline. But they also contain bundles of serotonin and co-factors that produce a hormone called kinin. Platelets that cluster in the blood vessels of the scalp can adhere together during stress or tension. This clumping bursts a certain amount of platelets, leaking serotonin which constricts the surrounding blood vessels and muscles. This raises the blood pressure by constricting the blood flow. The serotonin then enters the brain, passes the blood brain barrier, and surcharges the electrical impulses that regulate nerve impulses (through the reticular formation). This can cause the 'burst of anger' or tension headache.

As the platelets continue to break down, kinin leaks out. A powerful blood vessel widener, it has the reverse effect of serotonin, causing a rush of blood flow to the scalp. At the same time kinin zaps the pain sensors along the blood vessels throughout the neck and scalp, which gives rise to the throbbing headache.

Lymphocytes

The lymphatic system is the command centre of our immune system. It divides up into the primary system, thymus and bone marrow, and the secondary system, spleen, tonsils, lymph nodes, peyers patches, and appendix.

The immune fighting cells are produced in the primary system. These are the T-cells (thymus derived) and the B-cells (bone marrow derived). B-cells are responsible for producing anti-bodies. T-cells are the alert system identifying bacteria, fungi, parasites, and intracellular viruses, and thereby triggering cell-mediated immune response.

Range: 18-50% of total WBC
Mean: 30%

Levels below 18% indicate an exhausted immune system. In severe illness, low levels are associated with burns, AIDS-related complex, congestive heart failure, impaired lymphatic circulation, taking of immunosuppressive drugs and bone marrow suppression after chemotherapy, steroids.

Elevated levels above 50% are indicative of the same type of active viral infection, HIV, measles, mumps, chickenpox, influenza, hepatitis, infectious mononucleosis, cytomegalovirus (CMV) and lymphocytic leukaemia.

The absolute lymphocyte reading, 850-4100 cells/μL, can also appear on a blood panel and reflects the number of lymphocytes per cubic millimetre of blood.

Monocytes (Mononuclear cells)

These work in conjunction with neurophils in defending against infection, the difference being that these bacteria-swallowing cells (phagocytes) enter the blood stream not fully developed. Once they enter the tissues they grow, increasing their size as much as 4-5 times. Here they can stay for months, even years, until called upon to deal with bacteria.

Range: 0-9%
Mean: 5%

Lower readings are consistent with a healthy immune system.

Elevated readings above 9% are usually an indicator of a chronic or acute degenerative disease and tissue destruction. These can include bacterial infections, sub-acute infections, endocarditis (SBE), protozoal infections, hepatitis, ulcerative colitis, carcinomas and lymphomas.

The absolute monocyte reading, 200-1100 cells/μL, can also appear on a blood panel and reflects the number of monocytes per cubic millimetre of blood.

Neutrophils (Granulocytes)

Neutrophils, or phagocytes as they are also called because of their ability to engulf an antigen, operate like Pac-men in the blood stream, where they stay for 6-9 hours and then slip into the tissues where they live for a few days. The other common term used to describe organisms with this function is macrophages; they identify, kill and eliminate antigens (bacteria, viruses, fungi and toxins) from the body.

Range: 40-75%
Mean: 57%

Lower readings can indicate bone marrow depression due to radiation, chemical poisoning, i.e. benzene, chemotherapy and cytotoxic drugs (nucleoside analogues), overwhelming infections such as pneumonias, infectious mononucleosis, hepatitis and a large number of other drugs (including chloramphenicol, phenylbutazone, chlorpromazine, quinine). Hypoadrenalism, hypopituitarism, dialysis, liver disease and a deficiency of B-12 or folic acid will also lower levels. Elevated levels above 75% can be of a physiological nature, such as last trimester of pregnancy, surgery, excessive exercise, stress. Pathological elevations can be caused by bacterial infections, herpes, burns, carcinomas (cancer) and heart failure or inflammation (endocarditis). Metabolic disorders can include: rheumatic fever, rheumatoid arthritis, gout.

The absolute neutrophils reading, 1500-7800 cells/µL, can also appear on a blood panel and reflects the number of neutrophils per cubic millimetre of blood.

Bands

Bands are immature neutrophils (granulocytes) in the bloodstream at the time of sample.

Range: less than 5%

Readings below 5% indicate no active infection. Levels above 5% indicate an active infection.

Eosinophils

Another specialized granulocyte that functions to protect against allergic reaction and microscopic parasites. Identified because of its nucleus being stained with a red acid dye called eosin.

Range: 0-7%
Mean: 3%

Low levels, below 3%, are compatible with a healthy immune system although severely depressed readings can result from trauma, injury, burns or steroid drugs.

Elevated levels, above 7%, indicate allergic disorders: asthma, hay fever, food or drug reactions; parasite infection: amellasis, trichinosis, hookworm, roundworm; skin diseases: psoriasis, eczema, dermatitis, herpes. Other conditions can include collagen vascular disease, ulcerative colitis, pernicious anaemia, malignancy.

The absolute eosinophils reading, 50-500 cells/µL, can also appear on a blood panel and reflects the number of eosinophils per cubic millimetre of blood.

Basophils

Specific functions: releasing heparin into the bloodstream, which prevents blood coagulation, and facilitating the removal of trygycerides from the blood. Basophils also store histamine and are the largest source for blood histamine.[45] Histamine is a major neurotransmitter in the brain and throughout the autonomic nervous system (the self governing portion).[46] When released into the bloodstream, histamine can cause allergic and asthmatic reations.

Range: 0.3-2% (of total white count)

Mean: 1%

Low levels, below 1%, are sometimes found in people with rheumatoid arthritis, hyperactivity, and psychiatric problems.

Elevated levels, above 2%, can be related to drug reactions, parasitic infections, allergic and asthmatic reactions (inflammation and constriction of the lungs' air passages). High levels also have been associated with neurological and psychological disorders.

The absolute basophils reading, 0-200 cells/μL, can also appear on a blood panel and reflects the number of basophils per cubic millimetre of blood.

Anion / Cation Ratio (Anion Gap)

The anion gap reflects the acid/alkaline (anion, cation) balance in the blood at the time of the sample. Anions and cations are normally equal, maintaining an electrical neutrality in the blood. Sodium accounts for over 80% of circulating cations, chloride and carbon dioxide (CO_2) account for 85% of the anions. The gap between these levels represents anions not measured, such as phosphates, sulphates, organic acids (lactic acid, proteins), which determine types of metabolic acidosis.

Range: 8-14%

Mean: 10%

Low levels, below 8%, are rare, but may occur in bone marrow disease (multiple myeloma). Also drugs; antacids, diuretics or excessive sodium may decrease anion gap. A normal reading can be false positive if loss of body fluids (diarrhoea), re-absorption of sodium by kidneys causing retention of chloride create metabolic acidosis.

Elevated levels, above 14%, caused by accumulation of organic acids, sulphates or phosphates, can indicate: kidney failure, starvation, diabetes (insufficient production of insulin), alcohol intake, lactic acidosis, and drugs or chemicals that elevate sodium or decrease bicarbonate (CO_2).

Thyroxine (T4)

Thyroxine (T4) is an amine secreted by the thyroid gland in response to thyroid stimulating hormone (TSH) from the pituitary. T4 level is used to measure circulating thyroxine and as a thyroid diagnostic tool.

Range: 5-13.5 μg/dL (SI: 65–155 nmol/L)

Low levels below 5 suggest primary or secondary hypothyroidism. Liver disease, protein-wasting diseases, drugs, steroids, elevated sodium levels can all decrease T4.

Elevated levels are consistent with primary and secondary hyperthyroidism. Oestrogen and progestins can increase T4 readings, also pregnancy and severe illness.

Additional information on the immune system[47]

Without an immune system, as in the case of immuno deficiency conditions, the body quickly becomes overwhelmed by the micro-organisms (bacteria, viruses and fungi) that it is exposed to daily. We all have cancer every day:[48] antigens (foreign proteins) invade the body, feeding on healthy cells, and mutating them.

This is where the immune system begins to act, first by producing antibodies (immunoglobins) manufactured by the B-cells. When the B-lymphocyte identifies an antigen it grows and divides into plasma cells. The plasma cells then produce specific antibodies in large quantities that bind to the invading antigen and its clones. Some of these custom designed antibodies attach themselves to B-cells called memory cells, that remain in the system for future response should the body become exposed again to this particular antigen. The body does this by rearranging the DNA strands inside these cells to hold billions of different antibody types. This space saving strategy, like storing information on a computer disk, is called the immune system's humoral response because it takes place in the body's fluids (humoral immunity).

T-cells are the T-lymphocytes responsible for cell-mediated immune reactions, also called cellular response. Instead of producing antibodies to respond to antigens (intracellular viruses, parasites and bacteria), the T-lymphocytes produce helper cells that recognize antigens and trigger the release of the killer cells. The killer cells (lymphocytes) attach to the invading cell, killing it on contact by releasing a cell poison (cytotoxin).

T-cells such as T-helper cells can stimulate B-cells to respond to an antigen. T-suppresser cells turn off the immune response of the T-helper cells or the antibody producing B-cells once the invader has been killed.

If the balance of helper cells and suppresser cells, which is normally 1.8 helper to 1 suppresser, is altered by an immune-deficient condition, the T-suppresser cells can switch off the helper cells and B-cells. This allows antigens to go undetected throughout the body without a defence from the immune system. Once the condition exists, antigens that the body would easily deal with can become life threatening. (HIV, a very opportunistic virus, once it becomes active, creates this condition in the body.)

It is interesting to note that the B and T cells produced by bone marrow and the thymus do not have specific instructions or coding until they come into contact with an antigen. It is only then, for example, that specific antibodies or helper cells are produced.

Phagocytes (macrophages) are the clean-up crew. They are large white blood cells that are attracted to infection sites where they engulf and destroy antigens (micro-organisms). They will consume antigens attacked by B-cells and T-cells and eliminate them from the body.

These phagocytes (white blood cells) can also be a first line of defence. Snail like, they crawl along the blood vessels, passing through the blood vessel walls into the cells, looking for bacteria. They can engulf more than one bacteria and do so without it first being identified as a foreign particulate. These form the body's Pac-men.

One of the other ways phagocytes are mobilized is through the release of histamine from damaged cells. Once histamine enters the small capillaries in the tissue, the blood vessels swell, releasing a special protein stored in the crevices, which attaches to the antigen (microbe or invading bacteria) and kills it. Phagocytes respond to the histamine release by advancing toward the infection.

This is a difficult chapter to master; perhaps the most difficult in the book. But once you have mastered it, you will feel not only empowered, but also capable of fully understanding and participating in reprogramming your body for health. Believe me, I know; I have been there too.

13

Parasites and Bacteria

Any book on the body and how it works would not be complete without mention of parasites. Parasites are a factor of the human condition; our bodies can play host to almost 30 different parasites at any given time.

Parasites

We become infected from uncooked foods (especially uncooked meats), raw foods, contaminated water, pets, physical contact, etc. Once infected, eggs or cysts (flukes) then hatch in the body, developing into egg-producing factories.

This is not a phenomenon of the twentieth century; we have lived with parasites throughout our history. The difference is that today our immune systems which form the first line of defence to kill parasites are so compromised by the bombardment of pollutants that we are losing the battle. Backup systems like the liver which normally would kill eggs and their hatchlings, instead ends up playing host. The same thing happens to the pancreas, thymus and ultimately all areas of the body.

Parasites fall into two categories, protozoan (single cell organisms) and helminths.

Protozoan parasites include amoebas like Entamoeba hystolitica, responsible for hundreds of thousands of deaths every year globally from contaminated food and water by causing acute amoebic dysentery. Giardia lamblia is a jelly fish looking protozoan that is most commonly associated with water-borne contamination. Typically lodging in the small intestine, symptoms range from cramps, upset bowel, bloating, foul stool and gas. Symptoms usually develop slowly, over a week or more, with acute symptoms lasting up to three weeks.

The helminths include parasitic worms which develop after exposure to eggs in the intestinal tract and in the case of the Trichinosis larva, in the muscles. They include roundworms where eggs are found in contaminated meats, but are also spread by pets; tapeworms where eggs are found in contaminated meats, especially uncooked meat (steak tartar) and fish (sushi); and pinworms where eggs are spread by all sorts of contact, not only food but contaminated clothing and physical touch, and to which children are especially susceptible. There are also hookworms, whip worms, etc., the list is endless.

The real villains, however, are the fluke parasites and these come in a variety of shapes and sizes. The various forms include intestinal flukes (Fasciolopis buskii), liver flukes, pancreatic flukes, lung flukes (Paragonimus westermanii) and a number of animal flukes to which we are susceptible.

The immune system and parasitic infections

As mentioned earlier, the body has a capacity to eliminate flukes, but the ability is hampered by a weakened immune system. Once the immune system is overwhelmed, the parasitic flukes multiply through a number of ways. Strong chemical pollutants such as solvents dissolve the shells of the fluke eggs, allowing them to hatch in the body. Once this happens you are especially vulnerable. Through microscopic fissures or lesions in the intestinal lining, parasite eggs or hatchlings enter the blood stream. The liver, which at this stage would normally kill them, is also debilitated by the pollutant which then allows a reverse in its function to occur, wherein the liver actually plays host. From here the eggs or hatchlings start spreading throughout the body tissue.

The process from eggs to adult fluke is a multi step process which typically takes place outside the body. It is usually only the adult fluke that is found in the intestinal tract, laying eggs that are expelled through the bowel. If the eggs are allowed to hatch in the body, they complete their growth cycle in tissue and organs that have been chemically compromised.

The immune system tries to step in at this point and destroy them with engulfing (phagocytic) white cells. But if the immune system has been compromised by organic or inorganic contaminants and the eggs or hatchlings hide out in hard to reach organs like the liver, pancreas or even the brain, they go unchecked. Each egg produces spores that release dozens of additional eggs that develop into tadpole-like shapes that seek to attach themselves to tissue and form cocoons. Once again the various contaminants that may have released the eggs in the first place, or if in the intestinal tract, the body's own digestive fluids, will dissolve the cocoon, releasing the adult fluke. It is now capable of laying thousands of eggs daily, not only in the intestinal tract but throughout the body, and will continue doing so for years.

Steps involved in removing the contaminants affecting the immune system

The first step in preventing this process taking place in the body is to eliminate the causes. The list of organic and inorganic contaminants we are exposed to on a daily basis is frighteningly long.

It begins with chlorinated drinking or tap water. As you know it from Chapter 2, chlorine is one of approximately sixty chemicals (government regulated) that are added to tap water. Chlorine interacts with humic acid to produce trihalomethanes (chloroform being the most common) associated with several degenerative diseases.

Lead, cadmium, mercury, titanium, aluminium, tin, chromium, barium, antimony, strontium, benzene, propyl alcohol, propanol, isopropyl alcohol, isopropanol are just a few of the constituents or byproducts of the manufacturing process found in most products we use everyday. These include everything from deodorant, hair spray, lipstick, makeup, toothpaste, shampoo, soap, detergent, cleaning products, colognes, personal lubricants, shaving products, creams/moisturizers – almost all of our daily personal care products.

Read labels and look for ingredients such as propyl alcohol, propanol, isopropanol or isopropyl alcohol – RUN. Eliminate anything you have now with these or any of the previously listed ingredients. Propyl alcohol and benzene travel through the body at an incredible speed, and can be found in the thymus for example, within a minute of entry to the body.

Food products contaminated by solvents and contaminants include all commercially made cooking oils, all commercially made baking products, cereals, ice cream, packaged meats, sweets and packaged snacks; basically almost all commercially processed foods. Worthy of special note are beverages, which are laced with solvents, carbonated drinks, store-bought packaged juices, commercially produced bottled drinking water, decaffeinated coffees, infant formulas. All contain one or more of the following: methylene chloride, benzene, propyl alcohol, acetyl alcohol, methyl ethyl ketone, methanol, toluene, xylene, wood alcohol, acetone, carbon tetrachloride, decane, 1,1,1-trichloroethane, perchlorethylene (also used for dry-cleaning clothing). This list is endless.

Again you will not find these solvents on the list of ingredients, most are a result of the manufacturing process or residue of compounds used to clean or sterilize manufacturing equipment used in the process. This list does not even include pesticides (EDB, TCB and PCBs) which are inherent in all commercially grown crops and livestock, forming a residue on almost everything we eat and drink today.

I often hear comments from people about how their parents or grandparents lived into their 80s and 90s, and that their genetics alone should provide them with the same life span expectation. I usually answer this by asking them if they think their parents and grandparents were exposed to the quantities of contaminants (solvents, chemicals, pollution, pesticides and preservatives) that we are today and whether they believe that they would have experienced such long lives if they had.

The other areas of contamination are in our homes and workplaces. All cleaning, household, laundry, automotive products, emit toxic fumes absorbed by the body when it comes into contact with them. Remove all pesticides, mothballs, all chemicals used to destroy infestations, glues, aerosol sprays, room fresheners, carpet powders and sprays, spray starches, chlorine laundry bleaches (these are especially toxic), paint, solvents, gas cans. Once removed do not store them in your garage if it is attached to your house. The warm rising air of the house pulls the cooler air of the garage into the house and with it all the toxic fumes.

So we know that we have parasites, and we know that solvents, chemical pollutants, and pesticides destroy our immune system. How do we control the damage?

Side effects of common anti-parasitic drugs

First, of all the common drugs prescribed, not only are none effective in treating all parasites but they usually have side effects that can be as debilitating as the infection itself.

Flagyl (metronidazole) is used as an amoebicide and antibiotic treatment for amoebic dysentery, fungal and some bacterial infections. It can be effective for acute symptoms on a 3 day to 2 week dosage (most patients are over prescribed, amplifying side effects). Side effects include symptoms similar to infections: nausea, headache, dizziness, loss of appetite, occasional vomiting, diarrhoea, cramping and joint pain.

Atabrine (quinacrine) is a treatment for Giardiasis and tapeworm infections. Prescribed for 5 to 7 days, side effects include skin rashes, itching, headache, loss of appetite, cramping, diarrhoea, joint and muscle pain.

Yodoxin (iodoquinol) is used to treat amoebic infections and flukes (amoebic cysts). Often prescribed in combination therapy with Flagyl. Prescribed for 20 days, side effects include skin rashes, itching, headache, nausea, vomiting, stomach pain, diarrhoea, and thyroid gland enlargement. Prolonged use can cause blurred vision, eye pain, loss of muscular strength and co-ordination.[49]

Nutrients to enhance the body's immune control of parasites

There is no question that the body's most effective mechanism in controlling parasites is the immune system. And the way to ensure an immune response against them is to eliminate all immune suppressant conditions. This is where close scrutiny of not only what we are putting in and on our bodies is of vital concern, but also the contaminants we are exposed to in our home and work environment.

Only by detoxifying our bodies and our environment will we begin to feel better. Remember that the body has the ability to rid itself of solvents like benzene, propyl alcohol, etc., in less than a week after exposure stops.

There are a number of nutrients that can assist in neutralizing and eliminating pollutants and solvents from the body:

Flavanoids such as quercitin C, ellagic acid and chlorogenic acid have a protective effect against carcinogens like benzopyrenes, on a cellular and enzymatic level, reducing their bioavailability through the intestinal tract.[50]

B-vitamin B2 (riboflavin) helps the body in many ways. It maintains the mucosal barriers that defend against infection, and it is involved in the production of antibodies, formation of red blood cells, and in cell respiration. It is also very effective in neutralizing chemicals, specifically benzopyrenes in foods, by detoxifying them and preventing accumulation of benzene in the body.

B6 (pyridoxine) enhances the body's defences against pathogens. One of the most active nutrients involved in the body's chemical function, i.e. enzyme synthesis, fat and carbohydrate metabolism, hormone production, protein metabolism and neurotransmitter synthesis. It is also involved in antibody production providing protection against chemical antigens like benzene.

Glutamine is an ingredient for forming glutathione in the liver.[51] In its own right glutamine helps the body build muscle, is the major energy source for the gastro-intestinal tract and helps clear waste through the kidneys and liver. Its most important contribution is to the immune system, by increasing the production of phagocytes, the white cells that engulf and detroy bacteria and foreign material.[52]

Glutathione's role as the main scavenger of toxic oxidants works hand in hand with glutamine in helping to remove the detoxified waste from the body. Glutathione's ability to detoxify and prevent free radical damage is without equal. With adequate availability in the body, glutathione can detoxify almost all compounds and substances. Ranging from cigarette smoke, sun damage, air pollution, pesticides, heavy metals, radioactive chemicals, toxic gases and excessive alcohol consumption.

Beta Carotene is a potent anti-oxidant and quencher of singlet oxygen. It enhances immune function, prevents DNA damage, and it may counter the effects of benzopyrene exposure from cigarette smoke, industrial exposures (chemicals) and charcoal-broiled foods.[53]

Curcumin is a phenolic compound from spice turmeric. Curcumin exerts anti-carcinogenic activity by altering the activation and/or de-toxification process of carcinogen metabolism. In doing so it prevents chemical carcinogens like benzene and benzopyrene from reaching intracellular targets.[54]

Thioctic acid (lipoic acid) is a potent anti-oxidant, specifically inhib-iting free radicals caused by heavy metals like mercury, arsenoben-zoles, carbon tetrachloride, analine dyes, which it helps eliminate from the body. It also protects liver from toxicity due to poisoning. Thioctic acid interacts with glutathione to prevent lipid peroxidation, thus maintaining adequate tissue levels of free radical defences.[55]

Eliminating Parasites

Once we stop the bombardment of toxic mutagens and carcinogens like benzene, propyl alcohol, pesticides, PCBs, heavy metal, etc., we can begin to rebuild our immune systems to be able to destroy parasites. This is definitely a multi-step process; you can't rebuild cell mediated, humoral immunity and phagocyte response without this first step.

To attack, destroy and eliminate parasites from the body there are a number of potent parasite killers:

Garlic:	Raw garlic cloves on an empty stomach is an effective anti-parasite remedy. It contains many antibiotic properties. Deodorized garlic (missing some active ingredients) can be supplemented if you have a low tolerance for raw garlic.
Ginger:	Possesses significant anti-parasitic properties. Capsules of fresh ginger root may be used. Take on an empty stomach.
Grapefruit seed extract:	Effective anti-parasite agent.
Echinacea:	An important native American herb that inhibits parasites.
Raw pumpkin seeds:	Contains a compound that can kill intestinal worms.
Oil of Oregano:	Effective anti-parasite agent.

A formula to rid the body of parasites was conceived and promulgated by Dr H.R. Clark by combining three common herbs that have been used individually for years in the treatment of parasites. The combina-tion of the three herbs together works to rid the body of adult flukes and the developmental stages of at least 100 types of parasites. In doing so it rids the body of parasites on an intestinal, tissue and blood level. The formula included green-black walnut hull, wormwood (artemesia) and clove. The green-black walnut hulls and wormwood kill the adult flukes and other developing stages, and the clove kills the eggs. Dr Clark's formula consists of taking:

Black walnut hull tincture for 20 days, starting with one drop four times a day. On each consecutive day one drop is added until day 20 when you are taking 20 drops four times a day. From day 20 you take 20 drops once a day for three months. After three months, 30 drops once a day any two days a week (maintenance).

Wormwood Capsules for 14 days, starting with one capsule once a day. On each consecutive day one more capsule is added until day 14, then you take two more days of 14 capsules each day. Then you take 14 capsules two days a week continuously (maintenance).

Cloves (fresh ground) for 10 days, taking one capsule three times a day. On day two, take two capsules three times a day. On day three through ten, take three capsules, three times a day. After day 10, take three capsules once a day for three months. After three months, take three capsules and 2 days a week continuously (maintenance).

All three herbs to be taken on an empty stomach before meals.

This formula will rid the body of all parasites in five days and kill all eggs within three weeks. Afterwards the maintenance regime will deal with further re-infection. There is also a formula which includes all three herbs combined in a tincture form that I have found equally as effective as Dr Clark's protocol. Called Clarkia, it is available in a 60 ml dropper bottle (one month supply); 20-25 drops are taken three times a day before meals on an empty stomach.

Bacteria

Every day our bodies are bombarded with microbial contamination. These are one-celled organisms found throughout the body. Some of these bacteria are considered friendly bacteria, which the body uses to produce certain B vitamins, biotin, vitamin K, etc. But the delicate balance of friendly bacteria can be quickly overwhelmed by unfriendly bacteria. Our weakened immune systems prevent the humoral response where the antibodies produced by B-cells (lymphocytes) attach to the bacteria, killing and then engulfing them with phagocytic white cells.

Bacteria produce toxins that attack the body on a tissue and mucous membrane level, causing inflammation. In the case of the two most common infections, Staphylococcus and Streptococcus, they create very different symptoms. A Staph. infection is usually associated with food-borne illnesses and next to salmonella is the most frequent food poisoning. Symptoms include nausea, vomiting and diarrhoea within hours of ingestion. Also associated are skin ulcerations (pimples, boils, etc.), blood poisoning (Staphylococcaemica), infection in organs of the body (liver, kidneys, spleen, etc.), and pneumonia in lungs (most common bacterial cause of pneumonia). Strep. infections attack tissue, typically associated with throat infections, pharynx, tonsil infections; symptoms include high fever, chills, sweats, weakness, swollen glands and lymph nodes.

The common treatment for most bacterial infections is antibiotics. The problem with this is that the antibiotics kill all the body's friendly bacteria in the process. The loss of its defence against antibiotic resistant bacteria also results in yeast and fungus (Candida) attacks. Other drugs like cortisone, prednisone, antacids, and asthma medications also destroy the body's protective bacteria balance.

A recent newspaper article stated that half a century after the medical breakthrough of penicillin, antibiotics are losing their almost miraculous power to heal pneumonia, meningitis, tuberculosis and other dangerous infections. The antibiotics are being thwarted by 'Super Bugs' – bacteria with the ability to resist antibiotics.[56]

Antibiotics are the most over prescribed class of drug. Consequently, the bacterial microbes have developed resistance to antibiotics, and diseases we have not had to deal with for decades are returning in more lethal forms.

Remember also that antibiotics are widely used to treat cattle, pigs, poultry, and commercially raised fish, and to fatten livestock and prevent disease. Even people who do not take antibiotics are developing a resistance to them through the food supply.[57]

Other bacteria are becoming more prevalent in our daily lives. We are seeing outbreaks of major micro-biological threats. Some of these include:

• Listeria monocytogenes
• Salmonella
• Campylobacter
• E.-coli

Shigella and salmonella are two bacterias most commonly associated with food poisoning. Contaminated dairy products, fish (especially shellfish) and poultry will cause painful cramping/diarrhoea symptoms which are brought on within hours of ingestion. Shigella attacks the nervous system producing symptoms of nervous tension and irritability.

In many cases we can be infected and not be aware, as so much of our food and water is contaminated. But what we can do is reduce the bacterial load our body has to deal with daily and give our immune system the ability to dedicate its resources to repair and rebuilding. For this there are some natural antiseptics and antibiotics.

Honey

This is one of nature's most potent bactericides and antiseptics. Bacterial infections like Staph., Strep., and Candida, along with intestinal pathogens, Giardiasis, Shigella, salmonella, etc., are all killed by the powerful anti-microbial constituents of honey.

Since microbes (bacteria, parasites) are almost 90% water, honey's incredible osmotic capabilities (more than sea water) absorb their moisture,[58] thereby killing them.

This same osmotic effect plays a very important role in preventing fluid loss from diarrhoea. The sugars of honey create the osmotic pull, being 80% of its weight. Once in the bloodstream, they prevent water loss to the intestine and colon. Remember with diarrhoea, that it is not the intestinal tract that is losing water but the tissues and blood. Honey also helps retain electrolytes (discussed in Chapter 11) which provide the body's electrical charge.

Honey's organic acids are powerful germicides which, when applied topically to wounds and burns, can prevent infection and increase the healing process. Experiment with various skin conditions (rashes, acne, skin tears, bruises, boils, cysts, etc.) and note effects on infection and healing.

The important requirement is to be sure that the honey is pure, unfiltered and unpasteurized (unheated) for it to work. Processing reduces or destroys the enzymes, organic acids and antibiotics necessary to heal wounds and kill infection.

For topical use apply raw honey directly to the wound (cut, burn, surgical stitches, sores, etc.) two to three times a day. Cover area with gauze bandages and tape. Apply also before sleep.

For internal use – to treat food poisoning, intestinal flu, amoebic dysentery, and all parasite or bacterial induced diarrhoea – the dosage should depend on the severity of the condition. A minimum dosage for these conditions should be two tablespoons six times daily. A dosage of one-quarter of a cup four to six times daily may be needed for severe cases. Note however that Diabetics should not attempt internal use.

A daily maintenance dose of two tablespoons every morning can provide protection against parasites and bacteria.

Potent honey

New Zealand produces one of the most powerful antiseptic honies. Called Manuka honey, it has very potent anti-microbial properties. It contains aromatic acids which inhibit bacterial replication, and hydrogen peroxide which can kill bacteria on contact. (The brand name of a producer of this honey for export is *Comvita*.)

LDM *(Leptoaenia dissecta)*

Introduced to western medicine by the famous Dr E.T. Krebs, Jr. of the vitamin B15 and B17 fame, who made the statement that this single herb extract, 'Is destined to become one of the most important antibiotic herbs known to man!'. It is virustatic, bacteriostatic, and fungicidal, and can be used to treat Staph. and Strep. infections, respiratory and urinary infections, fungus infections, skin infections, and difficult viral infections. Note that a small percentage of people may be allergic to one of the oil factions and develop a harmless skin rash that may last for a few days; discontinue use if this happens.

Dioxychlor[59]

It releases nascent oxygen in the body, killing pathogenic bacteria (disease causing), germs, spores, mycoplasmas, viruses and fungi. Taken homeopathically under the tongue, goes directly into the lymph system.

Bee propolis[60]

The resinous substance bees collect from plants to help build their hives and keep it sterile. It has powerful antibiotic effects on all types of bacteria, viruses, fungi, and parasites. It stimulates the immune system by increasing the white blood cells (phagocytes) that engulf and digest micro-organisms. Propolis reduces inflammation of mucous membranes (throat, mouth), stomach and intestinal ulcers. Some of its active ingredients are cinnamic acid, anti-viral, caffeic acid, anti-cancer, and gallangian acid, a natural antibiotic.

Propolis is effective against Staphyloccus aureus, the bacteria resulting in blood poisoning, infections from wounds (surgical infections), and a type of pneumonia. Fighting the common cold or upper respiratory infections can be aided significantly by propolis' ability to prevent the replication of viruses. It can also be topically used for localized infections, cuts, burns, wounds, abrasions and bruises.

Tea Tree Oil[61]

This is another broad spectrum antiseptic, made from the leaves of the Australian tea tree. It has antiseptic effects on bacteria, viruses, fungi and parasites. For skin conditions, applied topically, tea tree oil stops infection and inflammation. It is also an effective antiseptic on burns, wounds, acne, rashes, eczema/psoriasis, fungal infections, insect bites, etc. Internally it can be used for gum infections, sinus infections, parasites, and bladder infections.

Tea tree oil has similar volatile molecules to alcohol, making it an effective inhalant for killing the air-borne bacteria that contribute to Strep. infections (lung, throat, sinus infections).

I advise people when they travel in public transport (trains, buses, airplanes, etc.) or if exposed to large crowds, to always carry some tea tree oil and a handkerchief. By placing a few drops on the handkerchief and inhaling every hour for a few minutes, air-borne bacteria and germs are killed before they have a chance to invade the body. This is especially important for people who work with the public daily and are thus constantly exposed to infection.

14

HIV

To illustrate how the information in this book can be applied to a condition. I have chosen as an example HIV.

This example hopefully will convince all reading the book, infected or not by the HIV virus, that our bodies have the ability to dominate a condition rather than have it dominate us. Indeed if this was not true, mankind would never have survived the scourge of plagues over the centuries.

Plagues, past and present, usually have their origins in bacteria. Almost all relate to a fast growing bacteria or virus brought on by unsanitary conditions, whether typhoid fever, malaria, or, the most extreme case, Ebola virus. How does this relate to HIV? First of all we should understand exactly what HIV is and how it infiltrates the body's cells.

HIV is a retrovirus,[62] which means it differs from other viruses in its ability to convert its RNA (ribonucleic acid), which carries its genetic information, into DNA (double-stranded deoxyribonucleic acid), the master molecule of life. For this unique conversion to take place it requires a special enzyme called reverse transcriptase, which acts as the catalyst. The virus attaches itself to the surface membrane of a cell, including the T4 helper cells – the foot soldiers of the immune system which identify antigens and trigger the release of killer cells. Once in the cell the genetic information of the HIV virus is transferred to a chromosome of the cell DNA. The now infected cell splits off a viral mutated copy of the original cell, often killing the host cell. The process is repeated as the viral copies go on to infect other healthy cells.

As the immune system's ability to defend the body is slowly compromised, conditions a healthy immune system would deal with quickly get out of control. Bacterial infections, viruses, parasites, environmental pollutants, etc., all play havoc with the body's operating systems as they now go unchallenged. And the reason they go unchallenged is that the HIV virus every day produces 100 million to one billion infected cells or new viral copies. The immune system also sends out an equal amount of virus fighting lymphocytes, which it draws from the body's ability to produce approximately two billion white blood cells daily.

Scientists believe that the virus' high rate of reproduction is what allows it to mutate and develop its resistance to drugs. This daily battle slowly wears down the immune system. It is also what makes HIV different from most viral infections, where the incubation period between infection and onset of disease symptoms is usually days or weeks. A common cold virus, for example, may have an incubation period of days before the onset of symptoms. The immune system mobilizes, dedicates the bulk of virus-fighting lymphocytes to battle the virus and usually health is restored relatively quickly.

HIV researchers now believe that the battle with the immune system starts from infection and not after a period of latency or dormancy. (This research was presented at the Second National Conference on Human Retroviruses and Related Infections in Washington, DC.) This would also explain why some people develop AIDS related conditions rela-⁺ively soon after being infected (within a few years) while others can go five, ten, twelve years before developing symptoms. And immune systems which are further compromised by factors such as life-style, diet, drugs, chronic health conditions, environmental pollutants, etc. will succumb soonest.

I have said for some years now that healthy people do not die from HIV. The basis for this claim lies in the maintainance of the immune system. Do not exhaust it. Think of it as your bank balance: if you were spending more than you were earning every day, sooner or later the accumulated deficit will bankrupt you.

The body produces only so many white blood cells daily, which are coded by the thymus for use by the body. If the immune system is overloaded because half of its resources are being used to fight the virus and the balance is battling the other factors mentioned above, little is left for the immune system to fulfil its primary function in the repair and rebuilding of the body.

It is at this moment that the body is most vulnerable. Opportunistic infections, whether bacterial, viral or parasitic, now easily gain a foothold. Free radicals from pollution, diet, and other environmental toxins run rampant through the body on a cell killing spree. A Staph. or Strep. infection which once would have been easy to fight off now becomes pneumonia or fever.

To make matters worse, most HIV infected patients are being treated with one or more anti-viral drugs. These include (AZT) ziduvudine, (D4T) stavudine, (DDI) didanosine, (DDC) zalcitabine or (3TC) lamivudine. All fall into the category of being 'nucleoside analogs', which target one viral enzyme and try to trick the virus into using the drug to build its DNA instead of the cells'. The problem with all of these drugs is they have very toxic effects on the body, and their effectiveness in reducing the viral load has a very short fuse – the virus can develop a resistance to or out-manoeuvre these drugs, often within a month to six months from their prescription. The current treatment has been to treat with a 'cocktail', a combination of three or four of these drugs; but this strategy has not prevented the virus from developing the same resistance within the same time frame.

The effects of these treatments are devastating to the body: the drugs are immune suppressant to begin with, and their negative effects are compounded by a debilitation of the body's chemistry.

One patient who came to me on the cocktail proudly announced that his viral load was very low, as if that was the good news. I said the bad news was that his body was in wasting mode, feeding on itself as a result of the toll the drugs had taken on his body. Every time his viral load would increase, he would be prescribed another drug – he was already on six when he first came to see me. The result of this treatment may be to keep the viral load down, but it also kills the patient. You do not cure a dog of fleas by putting the dog to sleep. I do not know what is served, least of all to the patient, if the treatment is as bad or worse than the disease.

The next generation of HIV treatment is a new class of drug therapy called protease inhibitors, a number of versions currently in clinical trials. Reports presented at the Washington DC conference stated that the protease inhibitors appear to be more potent than the nucleoside analogues at suppressing HIV replication and with fewer side effects. This has a very familiar ring to it; indeed the same has been said about AZT and every drug after it. Each time one was proved to be ineffective another was introduced, with the promise that when taken with the former they would become effective treatment. That has brought us to today, where one patient can be on as many as six different drugs. And already researchers are talking about using the protease inhibitors and nucleoside analogues together!

So where does that leave you? Trying to decide which poison is worse – the disease or the treatment.

If you have read this far, I hope you have realized that there are options. The subjects covered in the book can provide the road map for your well-being. In ten years of working with HIV I have not seen one person become symptomatic who applied the principles outlined in this book.

You understand now that the battlefront is the immune system, not the virus. If the immune system is able to operate at maximum capacity, it can dedicate the resources it needs to deal with the virus and do the necessary repair and rebuilding. But if the bulk of its resources are going to fight the factors of diet, drugs, bacteria, pollutants, and other health conditions, then there is no way it can do it all – especially with a casualty rate of HIV infected cells in the bloodstream of fifty percent every two days. A strong immune system, however, can reverse this percentage to the point where the virus is dominated and unable to gain an edge.

I am following up this book with a book on life threatening illnesses which will provide greater detail on this subject and more extensive treatment protocols for symptomatic individuals. But the information I want to impart here is the first step required for anyone infected or symptomatic. The fundamentals laid out in this book must be applied to build the foundation for recovery.

If you were going to start a course of exercise to get in shape, it would require going to the gym every other day. Over a period of months you would begin to realize the physical results. The same discipline and commitment must be applied here to achieve results. There is no overnight cure: it is going to require work each day to clean out and rebuild the body.

How do I start? What does it take?

The first thing I want you to do is get a thyroid test – the test I find most accurate is the Barnes basal temperature test. This test measures body temperature to determine thyroid function. If your body temperature is off as little as one or two degrees the consequences are serious. The body thinks it is losing heat and tries to conserve heat in the torso, which drops the temperature in the long bones (extremities) even more. The bone marrow of the long bones produce the bulk of our red and white blood cells. Production of these vital cells can be cut in half, which is critical in the case of white cells. If the daily white cell production of approximately two billion cells is cut in half, your immune system is debilitated before even tackling the HIV virus.

Next have a blood test, a full chemistry, and a complete blood count (CBC). Ask also for a thyroid-stimulating hormone (TSH) reading. The range for this reading is 0.7–5.3 mU/ml; you want to be close to a mean of 2.7–3.0. An increased level is indicative of hypothyroidism, a decreased level, hyperthyroidism. TSH is regulated by the pituitary gland, which triggers thyroid hormone production.

Over a third of the population is hypothyroid symptomatic; but these symptoms are often misdiagnosed and treated with antibiotics and other drugs that worsen the condition. Symptoms typically include:

- Cold hands and cold feet are the principal symptoms; the individual chills easily, and is unable to get warm.
- The feeling that every cold, flu, bronchial ailment going around was invented just for you.
- Fatigued, tire easily, go to bed tired, wake up tired, muscle cramps at night.
- Sensitive to touch, irritable; women can find sex uncomfortable.
- Headaches, depression.

These are among the most common symptoms; but the most accurate indicator is your white blood count. If it is down, this indicates a hypothyroid condition. And if your temperature test and TSH confirm this, the condition needs to be addressed as the first step to health. Your red and white cell production capacity has to be at its maximum.

I suggest that you check the iron level on your blood test, then check your total iron binding capacity (TIBC) reading. If both are low, especially the TIBC, either iron is low or the body cannot access what is available. This is where the cell salt (see Chapter 8) will come in handy, especially Ferrum Phosphoricum.

Specific nutrients to treat the thyroid and feed the endocrine system are:

A thyroid (thyrotropic) nucleoprotein complex (thyroid substance).
Tyrosine amino acid (see Chapter 6).
Vitamin C (ascorbic acid).
Molecular iodine.
Essential fatty acids – Alpha – linolenic acid, Oleic Acid (flax seed oil contains all), linoleic acid.
A complete range of neuropeptide glandular concentrates (for hypothalamus, pituitary, medulla, pineal, and all glands of the endocrine system).

All of the nutrients listed, other than tyrosine and vitamin C, which are taken on an empty stomach, should be taken with food, preferably lunch. The quality of the nutrients and the dosages are very important – check with a health care professional for your specific needs.

If your thyroid is functioning properly or you are addressing a hypothyroid condition, the next step is to limit the drain on the immune system.

Chronic conditions due to bacterial infections, Epstein Barr, Candida, parasites, and other viral infections (herpes, hepatitis) have to be brought under control. Environmental pollutants and chemicals must be eliminated where possible and neutralized where not (such as air pollution) before they have the opportunity to wreak havoc on the immune system.

There is no way the immune system can deal with all of these variables and the HIV virus and come out on top every day.

Food is the other major factor. The body has to fund hundreds of thousands of chemical reactions daily, all of which require fuel. Our diets provide the fuel or resources for our complex operating systems to function. Feed your body! Refer to Chapter 2 on food and food combining; then understand Chapter 3 on digestion: there is no point eating even the proper nutrients if the body is unable to access them.

Have a colonic (see Chapter 4). If the average person carries around over ten pounds of waste at any given time, you must remove these toxins. Waste is a tremendous drain on the immune system, especially if it is impacted on the colon wall, allowing toxins to be re-absorbed into the bloodstream. I cannot stress the importance of this enough.

Do your iridology worksheet (see Chapter 5), find out your constitutional strengths and weaknesses. Do you have a lymphatic rosary from poor hydration, nerve rings from stress? What shape is your colon in? How about a scurf rim from drug deposits? What shape are your heart, kidneys, liver, and other organs in? This is such an important step, you have to get to know your body better than anyone. Take Control!

Armed with your blood tests, refer to Chapter 12; go through your chemistry and blood count, establish where your strengths and weaknesses are. If you are at the low or high end of a range, the body is probably starving and deficient in specific nutrients, i.e. calcium, magnesium, iron, etc., or there is a metabolic problem brought on by infections, chronic conditions, pollutants, or any number of causes. The descriptions given (low or high end of range) will guide you, helping you to establish patterns for you to identify the reason for a low or high reading.

If there are deficiency related conditions refer to Chapter 6 on amino acids. We know that amino acids and the proteins they form are the nucleus of all cell structure. As such they form the second largest part of body weight next to water. Read the various descriptions for the individual amino acids, and cross reference against areas you have isolated on your blood work where there is a correlation.

Do the same thing with Chapter 8 on cell salts, which are vital constituents to healthy cells and tissue building. Cell salts can provide the most effective way of getting vital nutrients into the body in doses it can access and readily use.

Then go to Chapter 9 on homeopathy and Appendix A on the homeopathic first aid kit. Cross reference and become familiar with the various remedies for sudden, chronic or acute symptoms. These remedies, like cell salts, are extremely user-friendly to the body and can provide a consistent healing when taken properly. You are not going to reverse years of deficiency or conditions overnight. The repair and rebuilding process takes time, the body can only do so much in a given day. Homeopathy provides both remedies for the onset of symptoms (i.e. flu, fever, colds), and the constitutional properties for sustained healing.

Check Chapter 10 on electrolytes. If you are not drinking enough water, your electrolytes or batteries are going to be low. Your body needs a full electrical charge to operate efficiently.

Parasites and bacteria are the second major drain on our immune fighting ability, a toxic bowel being the first. Chapter 13 goes into detail about what these culprits do to the body and provides remedies for dealing with both. Parasites and bacteria unchallenged can drain away a major portion of your immune system every day.

The same principle applies to antigens from the air we breath, chemical fumes and exhaust, and many other pollutants. This is compounded by the mutagenic reactions (free radical forming) in the body through diet or exposure to mutagens.

As for cigarette smoking, drugs (illegal) or alcohol, their implication for the immune system speaks for itself. This knowledge I am sure you already have.

The cornerstone of my philosophy on dealing with HIV is that unless you can reduce the drain on the immune system you will not win the battle. The immune system is incredible and remarkable, and given a fighting chance it can sustain any challenge. But you must ensure that no undue or avoidable pressure is brought to bear on it. The protocols outlined in this chapter, and in detail throughout the book, will enable you to win the battle so many others have lost. Healthy people do not die from HIV.

15

Conclusion

The information in this book hopefully will serve as an owner's manual for your body. Having read the protocols and the basic operating principles of the body, use the reference guide to explore individual subjects in greater detail. There is a wealth of published information covering every area I have outlined, providing you with more detailed answers to any questions you may have.

Having said all that, I would like to finish the book in a more intimate way, speaking almost as if you had come to me for advice on how to take control of your health.

I want to start by saying that you must put aside all the programming you have hitherto received concerning your body. Open up your mind to the possibility that you can empower yourself to take control. No one knows your body better than you; no one can tell you how you feel. Your recovery to health depends upon your taking responsibility for your own health.

I often say to people that I feel most rewarded by working with people with life threatening conditions. The reason being that the motivation to change their life-style is greater. This is a decisive crossroads for most people; and for some, too decisive to be faced: 'What do I have to give up?' too often becomes 'What am I prepared to give up?' Because we have become conditioned to instant gratification, especially when it comes to our health, it is hard to convince most people that an aspirin is not going to reverse years of abuse and neglect. And if you are looking for an elixir of health or a panacea, you will not find it. To reprogramme the body takes a lot of patience and dedication. You are not going to reverse years of wear and tear just because you have decided to take supplements. As discussed throughout this book, a lot of people think because they are taking supplements they should instantly feel better. In fact we find that because they have no idea of what is involved for the body to benefit from whatever they are taking, they may as well not bother. Or may say, 'Well I'm taking supplements but I don't feel any better.'

You know now from reading this book that your body is a chemistry laboratory that works three shifts 24 hours a day, producing tens of thousands of chemical reactions. You know also that if the laboratory is bare, a lot of chemical reactions cannot properly take place. Once you add inherited genetic weakness and environmental conditions, you have the equivalent of replacing a car engine with a hamster on a treadmill.

Take a good look at yourself. Is your skin cross-linked? Wrinkled by the sun? Do you have digestive problems, heart problems, joint problems, nerve problems, etc.? The result of a chemistry laboratory mismanaged, neglected, even abandoned. Frankenstein's monster also began life with a collection of basically good parts; but at least he was not to blame for the way he turned out!

So do you have to become a biochemist? No; but what you need to understand is the principle of action and reaction, cause and effect, whatever you want to call it. For example, if you drink alcohol, that is an action; the reaction is its affect on the brain and other parts of the body. And we know now that we can neutralize those effects by re-stabilizing the body's chemistry with the B and C vitamins, anti-oxidants, etc., all the nutrients that alcohol affects directly or indirectly.

The choices available to you are varied; it really comes down to what you want to accomplish with your body. I assume that you want to accomplish something otherwise you would not be reading this book. You can have maintenance regimen, whereby you change little if anything in your life-style. Maintenance would include just neutralizing the effects of dietary and environmental reactions with supplementation. Another approach is to change certain dietary and environmental aspects of your life-style, in conjunction with supplementation for rebuild and repair. Or you can take the really radical step of changing not your life-style, but your life.

This approach requires most work because it requires getting in touch with your body's chemistry, and addressing its systemic, chronic or acute conditions. With a cursory knowledge, using some of the protocols outlined in this book, you can soon have a good working understanding of your body.

Iridology is an important diagnostic tool and will help to establish an initial diagnosis of your general condition. Find the colon around the pupil, look for the star burst of fine lines fanning out from the pupil that distinguish your constitution; look for nerve rings, the sodium ring, lymphatic rosary, scurf rim, fissures, and the organs they all correspond to. Look for inclusions and the corresponding parts of the body they may be impacting upon. Then have your blood work done.

Once you have compared your results with the laboratory values and referenced each category, you will obtain a window into your blood chemistry. This window allows you to start to identify deficiencies, metabolic irregularities, and overloads to the system. Most importantly becoming familiar with your blood panel allows you to establish the common threads that usually connect the problem areas. This will help you to isolate specific deficiencies, problems due to metabolic uptake, genetic malfunctions, and virtually impaired immune system activity. A simple blood panel will provide you with a detailed picture of what is going on chemically in your body.

Then you apply the three basic principals of life: respiration, assimilation and elimination. The air we breathe in most metropolitan areas is approximately 20% (or as little as 12%) oxygen. This oxygen depleted air, already contaminated by pollutants, reacts with reactive oxygen species. Hydroxyl radical (OH) initiates most atmospheric and pollutant-driven conversions. These include nitrogen oxide from the combustion of engines and power plants and sulphur dioxide emissions due to industrial pollution. Not only are we breathing oxygen-depleted air, but air that is loaded with free radicals that damage cells and organs.[63] Ordinary city air on a typical day can contain over a billion hydroxyl radicals per lung full of air!

Too much oxygen, if your anti-oxidant levels are deficient, can lead to increased free radical activity. So it becomes extremely important, especially in hyper-oxygenating the body, to make sure your anti-oxidant levels are high. I use and recommend a number of oxygenators such as sodium chlorite bonded with sodium carbonate, and wheat grass which has naturally occurring anti-oxidants.[64] All of these I have discussed in previous chapters. The important fact about oxygen is that we need it – and a lot of it. At adequate levels, oxygen stimulates our body's anti-oxidant properties. Too little oxygen debilitates the free radical fighting ability, but not the free radical forming ability. So the solution is the obvious one: anti-oxidants! anti-oxidants! anti-oxidants!

I am struggling to find the words to explain most powerfully just how important is the assimilation of nutrients. The best way is to tell you something that I experienced recently. I have begun using a laboratory in Texas called *Specta Cell Laboratories* which does essential metabolic analysis (EMA) testing, a nutrient blood analysis to determine how well nutrients are working at a cellular level. (They also perform an anti-oxidant function test.) Their methodology is to test a growth response of lymphocytes to a particular nutrient, a serum-free, protein-free, chemically defined medium they call CFB1 1000. Having taken mega doses of supplementation over the last 14 years, I was very curious about my own nutrient levels. Needless to say I was thrilled when excellent results came back. There were a few nutrient levels that could be higher, but for the most part I had achieved optimum results.

This illustrates my whole attitude towards health and healing, that unless we have adequate reserves of nutrients available to the body, disease symptoms develop, aging is triggered and accelerated and organ atrophy begins.

Government studies (Health and Nutrition Examination Survey) identified 70% of the American population to be at risk from the clinical impact of long term dietary deficiencies. Private research institutes, like *Spectra Cell*, found that 81% of all patients tested were deficient in essential nutrients. In the latter group, 53% of those tested were taking some form of supplementation. What was wrong?

What was and is wrong is that we are not assimilating the nutrients taken into our body. As discussed in Chapter 3 on digestion, nutrients enter our digestive tract (for purposes of illustration) the molecular size of golf balls. Our digestive system has to reduce that size down to the size of a pea. This requires thousands of enzymes, each coded to address different substances. We know already that this system is easily sabotaged by improper food combining, over hydration (water), diluting hydrochloric acid and enzymes, and not producing enough hydrochloric acid or enzymatic action even to begin the process.

Over the years I have heard hundreds of people say that they are taking vitamins and do not feel any better; and, if anything they feel worse. By asking a few simple questions as to diet, food combining habits, types of supplementation, and when they are taking the supplements, it becomes quite clear why they are not deriving any benefit from them, and even receiving an adverse reaction.

Typically people will take supplements that require digestion on an empty stomach, which can upset the stomach. Then they will take the water soluble supplements that require no digestion, but need to be taken on an empty stomach, with food. Finally, they will take vitamins, minerals and herbs with a meal, which they will complete with a simple carbohydrate (dessert), thus stopping digestion in its tracks. In each case, taking supplements was a total waste of time and money, for little or nothing was assimilated.

Unless we are prepared to accommodate the body's operating systems for nutrient retrieval and utilization, all we are doing is feeding our appetite and not our body. I cannot stress this simple fact enough: we are nothing but tens of thousands of chemical reactions every day, and without the resources to fund these chemical reactions we have not only accelerated the aging process but opened the door to disease.

The body eliminates through a number of pathways: the colon, the kidneys, lymph system, lungs, and skin. All of these require maintenance to function efficiently. Diet also plays an integral role. Our body was designed with this incredible system of converting nutrients into fuel and eliminating waste and toxins. But it is a delicate system with all sorts of checks and balances.

The skin, for example, has over two million sweat glands, each with minute tightly coiled tubes that could extend four feet. The approximately eighteen square feet of skin in the average adult can generate 3 to 4 quarts of sweat during strenuous exercise and about a quart or more in daily activity. Through sweat we eliminate sodium, potassium, milk sugars, and toxins eliminated from the blood.

The lungs eliminate every day the equivalent of two heaped table-spoons of solid particulate matter (bacteria, metals, carbon, glass, tar, acids, dust, pollen, smoke, rubber, etc.).

The kidneys control electrolytes, eliminate uric acid (a byproduct of protein metabolism), control the acid/alkaline balance of blood, process up to 3,500 gallons of water daily, and produce hormones that release red blood cells, vitamin D and help to regulate blood pressure.

The lymph system is our back-up route for nutrients, especially proteins, fats, and particulate matter too large to be re-absorbed into the capillaries, which is carried away from the tissue spaces. Its essential function is to remove proteins and excess water from the interstitial spaces (tissue) otherwise cells would drown.

The colon is a dehydrator, eliminator, and one of the major contributors to our overall well-being. When functioning properly there is nothing man has created that can match it. When malfunctioning, which is the case in the majority of the population, it is the largest contributor to disease in the body. Auto-intoxication through recycling toxic waste into the blood stream; impacted waste accumulation that becomes carcinogenic (cancer causing); Candidiasis; and bad food combining, causing food to remain in the digestive tract three times its normal time. All of these factors make the colon our major focus in a maintenance program that includes colonic irrigation and friendly bacteria balancing.

If these three principals of life – respiration, assimilation, and elimination – are applicable to our very existence, how do we begin a maintenance program that services the over 100 trillion living cells that make up our body on a given day?

I began this book by remembering the very first health food store I consciously walked into, and how I felt overwhelmed by all the different products. In time I came to realize that the reason for all the different vitamins, minerals, herbs, etc. was because the body utilizes and needs all of them. When you take just one of the body's operating systems and look at the chemical interactions necessary for its function this becomes immediately apparent.

With that appreciation also comes the realization that very few people are even getting close to their body's nutrient requirements. The Recommended Dietary Allowances (RDAs) set by the Food and Nutrition Board states that the general population consuming food containing the RDA's essential nutrient requirements have not been known to develop any nutritional deficiency diseases related to nutrients. However, there are over 100 million adults in this country suffering from allergies, arthritis, rheumatism, diabetes, hypertension, etc.,[65] which does beg the question, when is a disease not a dietary related disease?

My advice to you is to start feeding your body now! Today! You are no longer intimidated by the prospect. You have a working guide in your hand with plenty of references for additional information. Start using it! If you feed your body today you are fighting back. Do not emphasize on what you might have to give up; emphasize on what you know you will gain: a long and healthy life. Knowledge is power: if you know that you are doing something that has an adverse reaction on the body, then at least neutralize its effect by giving your body the antidote. Stop aging, stop disease; it is all within your reach – literally, the reach you make for your supplements every day.

Play chemistry with your body; use some of the protocols described in this book; try them for a month even, and see if there is a difference in how you feel. This is such an exciting time for you to be embarking upon or expanding your knowledge in reprogramming your body for health. There has never been such an exciting array of products available as there is today or so many incredible people doing such great things in this area of research. Be the beneficiary of the advances that are occurring every day.

Take control.
Be healthy.
Be happy.
And spread the word.

Appendix

Your Homeopathic First Aid Kit

These are remedies to have on hand for acute (sudden onset, short lived) conditions. I have listed them as individual remedies, but most if not all come as combination remedies. The theory behind combination remedies is that symptom patterns may be different in each of us. The mixing of various remedies that treat similar symptoms of a condition ensures that one or more of the remedies will effect a cure. Each single remedy can treat well over a hundred different symptoms, but are primary cures for specific conditions on a descending scale.

It is my belief that homeopathy works on a molecular level, not only in the cells and tissues but also the body's immune system antibody memory. By this I mean for conditions like flu, viruses, infections, any condition the body has developed and to which it has stored an antibody blueprint (in the DNA stands – refer to Chapter 12 on the immune system). What you are trying to achieve is a match, the principles of homeopathy law of similars, 'like cures like'. An immune response stimulated by triggering the antibody that effects a cure.

Combination remedies are used to cover a large range of variables; trying to find a match for a particular symptom could be like looking for a needle in a haystack. But when the match is made, the cure begins immediately and the symptoms disappear.

The remedies given below should be administered in doses of 30C potencies for acute conditions and 6-30X potencies for chronic conditions. There are a number of protocols for taking homeopathic remedies. Typically 3–5 pellets are taken sublingually (under the tongue) on an empty stomach, and not having drunk any fluids for 15 minutes before or after. As the pellets dissolve, the remedy is absorbed throughout the blood vessels into the bloodstream. Another way is to dissolve one or two pellets in a glass of distilled water to be sipped throughout the day. Upon contact with the oral cavity the diluted remedy stimulates a nerve response in the tongue, thus triggering an immune response. The third application is topical, where the remedy is absorbed through clean skin. This treatment would be used in cases of burns, sprains, bruises and muscle injuries.

Arnica Montana

Use immediately after a tissue trauma such as sprains, bruises or muscle fatigue brought on by physical exertion. It brings about incredible relief and is very effective in treating old injuries to muscles and connective tissue. It will also reduce and localize blood loss due to sudden traumas, preventing oxidation due to haemoglobin leaking into tissue (black and blue marks). Very important in treating head injuries and strokes.

Aconite

Provides relief for conditions or symptoms that come on suddenly, such as fear or a fright where the adrenaline is pumping and the nerves are sensitive. Or flu or fever symptoms, brought on by exposure to cold dry wind and a resulting chill. Symptoms include headaches, dry sore throat, flushed face, sensitivity to touch and sometimes nausea and vomiting. Aconite is effective, if taken immediately, in eliminating these symptoms overnight.

Apis

Deals with sudden inflammations that have burning or stinging characteristics. Also a swollen sore throat, eye infections, urinary infections and hives brought on by allergic reactions. Made from ground-up parts of the honey bee, making it effective as an antidote to bee and wasp stings.

Arsenicum

Don't leave home without this one! Arsenicum is a most effective remedy for food poisoning brought on by, for example, Salmonella in chicken, E. Coli bacteria in meat, and amoebic dysentery from untreated drinking water. Also an effective remedy for late night coughing, dry, wheezing, burning chest, asthma attacks and breathing difficulties. Good for cold symptoms which involve a lot of mucous discharge, coughing and bronchial constriction.

Belladonna

Use for head complaints that come on suddenly and with intensity. Symptoms include flushed redness with swelling and burning sensation, throbbing headache, and ear infections aggravated by cold and touch. Belladonna provides a restful sleep, and alleviates dryness of mucous membranes that lead to coughing.

Bryonia

For the treatment of cold and flu symptoms that begin slowly producing that tired, fuzzy head, ache-all-over feeling. These symptoms develop into painful headaches (made worse by movement), sore joints and muscles, and bronchial dry coughing that strains the chest.

Carbo Veg.

Provides relief of cramping pain from gas build up in the intestinal tract. Symptoms also include belching, heartburn, flatulence with a bloated feeling. Bad food combining, over-indulgence or drinking too much fluid with meals, preventing digestion, can all be contributory factors.

Chamomilla

Very effective for people very sensitive to pain. Children especially can gain relief from teething, ear infections, colic, and other childhood maladies that cause irritable behaviour. Women gain relief during menstrual periods. Also used in treatment of symptoms resulting from caffeine and narcotics withdrawal.

Drosera

For that irritating dry cough that usually hits between 12 and 3 am and accompanied by tickling irritation of the larynx and back of the throat, that increases the frequency and intensity of the cough and sometimes the sensation of not being able to catch your breath.

Ferrum Phosphoricum

There is that initial flush, like coming into a warm room from out in the cold feeling, accompanied by aching joints and muscles. A fever develops, throbbing headache, sweating and thirst for water. Ferrum Phosphoricum can be very effective in the early stages when these symptoms first appear. Also useful in the treatment of ear infections and nose bleeds.

Gelsemium

Also a flu and cold remedy, especially when the symptoms develop slowly. These symptoms usually begin with congested head and headaches, followed by a feeling of exhaustion, total lack of energy, aching

Appendix

and a need to lie down and be still. They are sometimes accompanied by involuntary urination or defaecation.

Hepar Sulphuris

For cold and flu symptoms that include a lot of mucous discharge both through coughing and sinus drainage. Also where the body is sensitive to cold, and you can't seem to get warm and also a general sensitivity to touch. Other symptoms include sweating, swollen glands, skin eruptions and sore throat.

Ipecacuanha (Ipecac)

Provides relief of nausea with sudden onset, which can include vomiting that does not relieve nausea. Also good for head colds that congest the sinuses, and then move into the bronchial passages. Usually accompanied by a dry hacking cough with mucous that is difficult to expel. Useful in the treatment of colic and diarrhoea in infants.

Kali Bichromicum

For people who are always clearing their throat of mucous (catarrhal), which constantly builds up at the base of the tongue. Those suffering from recurring sinusitis can also benefit from relief of sinus pressure and chronic mucous build up in sinuses. Also used for sharp severe shooting pain in isolated areas throughout the body that appear and disappear quickly.

Ledum

Used to treat flesh wounds, where the skin has been broken. Effective treatment for haematomas, haemorrhages under the skin, such as black eyes or where the tissue has been damaged and blood has leaked into it. Helps speed up the re-absorption of fluids and reduce swelling. Very important remedy to have on hand to deal with insect bites.

Mercurius

For symptoms of sensitivity to both heat and cold. Also excessive perspiration, aching joints, chills and mucous discharge. Other conditions can include toothaches and gum disease, swollen or inflamed glands and foul odours of sweat, breath, flatulence, and stools. A general weakness, lack of appetite and restlessness can also be symptoms.

Nux Vomica

Can provide relief if you have eaten too much or indulged in bad food combining, spicy foods, alcohol etc., especially if indigestion is accompanied by heartburn, headaches, bloating and gas. Also used to treat individuals who are stressed out, irritable, unable to relax or sleep properly. Effective in treatment of pre-menstrual conditions.

Phosphorus

For individuals who experience general tiredness and sensitivity to noise, touch, smell, cold and who become dizzy if they rise too quickly and experience headaches that are throbbing and congestive. Also effective for relief of chest colds, especially those with a heavy bronchial chest and dry rasping cough, and laryngitis that leads to voice loss, particularly in the evening.

Pulsatilla

On a psychological level used to treat nervous, changeable, moody behaviour, individuals who need a lot of attention or comfort. On a physical level effective for head colds and sinus discharge for digestive disturbance from illness or over eating rich foods, and for eye, ear and nose conditions, such as styes, nose congestion, and nose bleeds.

Rhus Toxicodendron

A remedy for relief of joint, ligament, tendon and skin conditions brought on by over exertion, or exposure to cold damp weather. Can be associated with fever type headaches where the head is sensitive to touch and movement. Used to treat skin rashes and eruptions, such as fever cold sores and poison ivy.

Silica

Acts on the more organic constituents of the body such as joints, bones, glands, skin and mucous membranes. Also a component of the nervous system. Effective in removing infection (pus), leaked blood products from injury or fluid from swelling joints and tissues, by eliminating them through the lymphatic system. Especially useful not only as a constituent in rebuilding connective tissue, but also in removing (through the lymphatic system) the urates produced by rheumatic and arthritic conditions that destroy connective tissue. Effective treatment for enlarged lymph nodes, inflamed glands, dry cracked skin, lips, and nose bleeds. Very important in maintaining flexible arteries, preventing cardiovascular disease. Silica counteracts or neutralizes the effects of aluminium on the body, which is linked to Alzheimer's disease.

Sulphur

Acts as the body's antiseptic, both internally and externally. Sulphur springs date back to the Romans as treatment for flesh wounds and skin diseases. Psoriasis, eczema, and dermatitis all benefit form sulphur's anti-bacterial properties. Internally sulphur kills bacteria in the bloodstream. Because of its anti-oxidant properties it protects the cells from toxic antigens like pollution and powerful mutagens like radiation. It also stimulates the liver's bile secretions and absorption of other minerals. Sulphur is a constituent of haemoglobin and all body tissue and is needed for the synthesis of collagen, which provides the elastin in skin, hair, and nails.

Glossary

ACETALDEHYDE: A damaging mutagen and carcinogen found in air pollution, cigarette smoke, alcohol.

ACUTE: A condition arising suddenly and manifesting intense severity, usually accompanied by pain and inflammation, but lasting only a short time. (Homeopathic definition.)

ADHESIONS: Tissues in the body stuck together.

ALDEHYDES: Very reactive free radicals causing mutagenic and carcinogenic reactions in the body. Chemicals and peroxidized fats being the biggest contributors.

ALIMENTARY TRACT: Gastro-intestinal tract – the gut.

ALLERGEN: A substance that brings about an allergic reaction.

AMINO ACID: Building blocks of protein that consist of amino basic group (nitrogen and hydrogen) and acid of carboxyl group (carbon, oxygen and hydrogen).

ANAEMIA: A condition resulting from an unusually low number of red blood cells or too little haemoglobin in the red blood cells.

ANAEMIA, PERNICIOUS: Anaemia caused by a vitamin B12 deficiency.

ANAEROBE: A germ or bacteria that can multiply without an oxygen supply.

ANTAGONIST: Refers to nutrient interactions that inhibit one another. Copper and zinc are antagonists (zinc inhibits copper absorption), while calcium and vitamin D are agonists (vitamin D helps to promote calcium absorption).

ANTIBIOTIC: Medication that helps the body fight infection by neutralizing or destroying bacteria.

ANTIBODY: Proteins produced by B cells of the body in response to an offending agent, viral, bacterial or cancer.

ANTIGEN: Any substance that brings about the production of antibodies. Antigens may be externally introduced or formed within the body.

ANTI-OXIDANT: A substance that slows oxidation (see oxidation). Examples include vitamins C and E, the minerals selenium and germanium, superoxide dismutase (SOD), coenzyme Q10 catalase, and some amino acids.

ARCUS SENILIS: A white/yellow arc around the periphery of the upper section of the iris which often leads to the formation of a cholesterol ring.

ARTERIOSCLEROSIS: A common arterial disorder. Characterized by calcified yellowish plaques, lipids, and cellular debris in the inner layers of the walls of large and medium-sized arteries.

ARTERY: Blood vessel that carries blood away from the heart to the organs, glands, and tissues.

ASCENDING COLON: The section of large intestine on the right side of the body rising from the appendix to the liver.

ATP: Adenosine triphosphate, an energy molecule released and broken down, on demand, to meet the body's energy needs.

AUTO-ANTIBODIES: A self-produced antibody acting against a person's own body.

AUTO-ANTIGENS: Any substance within our own body that brings about an antibody reaction that attacks its own cells.

AUTO-IMMUNE DISEASE: Occurs when the body's immune system reacts to and damages its own tissues and organs. Examples include multiple sclerosis, rheumatoid arthritis, systemic lupus, Bright's disease, and diabetes.

AUTONOMIC NERVE WREATH (ANW): The wreath seen around the pupil usually situated approximately a third of the distance between the pupil and outer edge of the iris. It indicates the condition of the autonomic nervous system and also the shape of the large and small intestines.

BACTERIA: Microscopic germs. Some bacteria are 'harmful' and can cause disease, while other 'friendly' bacteria protect the body from harmful invading organisms.

BETA-CAROTENE: A derivative of vitamin A. Widely accepted today as a cancer preventative.

BILE: A substance released by the liver into the intestines for the digestion of fats.

BLOOD-BRAIN BARRIER: This is a cellular barrier which prevents certain chemicals from passing from the blood to the brain. Many amino acids and substances are blocked from entering into the brain readily without a transport system.

BLOOD COUNT: The number of red and white blood cells and platelets in a sample of blood.

BUTYLATED HYDROXYTOLUENE (BHT): An artificial preservative added to oils to slow down their deterioration; it replaces vitamin E, which is removed during oil processing.

BUTYRIC ACID (BA, 4:0): A short-chain (4-carbon) saturated fatty acid found in butter. BA is beneficial to normal intestinal bacteria.

CAPROIC ACID (6:0): A short-chain (6-carbon) saturated fatty acid found in tropical oils and to a small extent in medium-chain triglycerides (MCTs).

CAPRYLIC ACID (8:0): A medium-chain (8-carbon) saturated fatty acid found in tropical oils and in medium-chain triglycerides (MCTs).

CARCINOGEN: Any agent that is cancer-causing.

CATARACT: A disease of the eye in which the crystalline lens of the eye becomes partially or totally opaque.

CELL: All living tissues are composed of cells, which are very small complex units consisting of a nucleus, cytoplasm, and a cell membrane.

CELL-MEDIATED IMMUNITY: Types of immune reactions that involve T-cells.

CELL MEMBRANE: A double layer of fatty material (phospholipids) and proteins that surrounds each living cell of all organisms.

CHOLESTEROL: A crystalline substance, consisting of various fats, that is naturally produced by all vertebrate animals and humans. Cholesterol is widely distributed and manufactured in the body and facilitates the transport and absorption of fatty acids.

CHOLESTEROL RING: (also called sodium or mineral ring) A white, or yellowish-white ring around outer edge of the iris indicating hardening of the arteries (arteriosclerosis) caused by excess sodium/calcium deposits and high levels of cholesterol.

CHOLINE: A pseudo-vitamin involved in the metabolism of fats and in nerve function, and found in lecithin (phosphatidylcholine).

CHRONIC: Long-standing condition seen as a dark discolouration in the iris.

COENZYME: A heat stable molecule that must be associated with another enzyme for the enzyme to perform its function in the body. It is necessary in the utilization of vitamins and minerals.

COFACTOR: The part of an enzyme that is usually a mineral or trace metal important for the activity of the enzyme.

COLD-PRESSED: A method used to process oils from food without heat to preserve the nutrients.

COLITIS: Inflammation of the colon.

COLON: Term for the large intestine (ascending, transverse and descending).

CONGENITAL: A condition existing from birth, although not necessarily hereditary.

CONSTITUTION: The physical and psychological make-up of a person, revealing that person's general state of health and inherent strengths and weaknesses.

CROSS-LINK: Bonds that form across molecules and result in complex molecular structures. Also, bonds that make tissues more rigid, leading to aging.

CYTOTOXIN: A poison that attacks various tissue and organs and is produced by introducing foreign cells.

D, L and DL: Amino acids occur in D and L forms. The D form rotates light to the right, while L form rotates to the left. When the amino acid occurs in DL, it's a mixture of D and L.

DEGENERATIVE STAGE: The final stage of degeneration and tissue breakdown, seen in the iris as black discolourations.

DEOXYRIBONUCLEIC ACID (DNA): The genetic material that carries the instructions for most living organisms.

DESCENDING COLON: The section of the large intestine on left side of body going down from near the spleen to the rectum.

DETOXIFICATION: The process of reducing the body's toxic build-up of various poisonous substances.

DIHOMOGAMMA-LINOLENIC ACID (DGLA): A fatty acid, the second omega 6 derivative; made from GLA; DGLA is the parent of hormone-like series 1 prostaglandins which have many beneficial effects on health.

DIURETIC: Increases urine flow, causing the kidneys to excrete more than the usual amount of sodium, potassium, and water.

DNA (DEOXYRIBONUCLEIC ACID) The substance in the cell nucleus that genetically codes amino acids and their peptide chain pattern, and determines the type of life form into which a cell will develop.

ELECTROLYTE: A chemical substance with an available electron in its structure that enables it to transmit electrical impulses when dissolved in fluids.

ELIMINATIVE CHANNELS: Five main channels for elimination of toxic waste from the body are lungs, bowels, kidneys, skin and lymph.

ENDEMIC: Used to refer to a disease that constantly occurs in any particular geographical region.

ENZYMES: Very large proteins that activate certain reactions in the body to form specific substances.

EPSTEIN BARR VIRUS (EBV): A virus that causes infectious mononucleosis and that is possibly capable of causing other diseases in immunocompromised hosts.

ESSENTIAL FATTY ACIDS: Substances that the body cannot manufacture and therefore must be supplied in the diet. See fatty acids.

ETHYLENE DIAMINE TETRAACETIC ACID (EDTA): A chelating (clawlike) molecule used to remove heavy metals and calcium from the human body, it is one way of treating heavy metal toxicity and atherosclerotic deposits in arteries.

FATTY ACID: An acid derived from the series of open chain hydrocarbons, usually obtained from the saponification of fats.

FATTY ACIDS: Nutritional substances found in nature (fats and lipids), which include cholesterol, triglycerides, fatty acids, prostaglandins, and stearic, palmatic, linoleic, eicosapentanoic (EPA), and decohexanoic acids. Important nutritional lipids include lecithin, choline, gamma-linoleic acid, and inositol.

FREE RADICAL: A free radical is an atom or group of atoms that has at least one unpaired electron. Because another element can easily pick up this free electron and cause a chemical reaction, these free radicals can effect dramatic and destructive changes in the body. Free radicals are activated in heated and rancid oils and by radiation in the atmosphere, among other things.

FUNGUS: One-celled organisms belonging to the plant kingdom. Its members contain a number of species including Candida albicans, which are capable of causing severe disease in immunocompromised hosts.

GASTRO-INTESTINAL: Pertaining to the stomach, small and large intestines, colon, rectum, liver, pancreas, and gall bladder.

GLAND: An organ that excretes materials and manufactures substances not needed for its own metabolic function.

HAEMOGLOBIN: A molecule of which iron is an essential component. Necessary in the red blood cell's transport of oxygen.

HELPER T-LYMPHOCYTE: A lymphocyte subtype active in the process and stimulation of immunity. This cell is the one principally infected and killed by the AIDS virus.

HERING'S LAW OF CURE: Healing proceeds from within out, from the top down, in reverse order and from vital organs to less vital organs.

HISTAMINE: A chemical in the body tissues that constricts the smooth bronchial tube muscles, dilates small blood vessels, allows fluid leakage to form itchy skin and hives, and increases secretion of stomach acid.

HOMEOPATHIC: A type of drugless therapy based on the theory of 'like cures like'; opposite of allopathy where drugs are used.

HOMEOPATHY: A system of medicine based on the belief that the cure of disease can be effected by minute doses of substances that, if given to a healthy person in large doses, would produce the same symptoms as are present in the disease being treated. Homeopathy employs natural substances in small doses to stimulate the body's reactive process to remove toxic waste and bring the body back into balance.

HORMONE: An essential substance produced by the endocrine glands that regulates many bodily functions.

HOST: An organism in which another micro-organism lives and from which the invading micro-organism obtains nourishment.

HUMORAL IMMUNITY: Various immune-related substances and actions generated by the bodily fluids.

HYDROCHLORIC ACID (HCl): An inorganic acidic compound, excreted by the stomach, that aids in digestion.

HYPERACID STOMACH: Excess HCl (hydrochloric) acid in the stomach zone seen as a bright white discolouration (acute) or a white/silver halo (sub-chronic) in stomach ring in the iris.

HYPOACIDITY: Lack of acid and diminished function.

HYPOCALCAEMIA: Abnormally low calcium levels in the blood.

IMMUNE SYSTEM: A combination of cells and proteins that assists in the host's ability to fight (i.e. resist) foreign substances such as viruses and harmful bacteria. The liver, spleen, thymus, bone marrow, and lymphatic system are inter-related in the immune system's normal function.

IMMUNODEFICIENCY: An immune reaction deficiency involving antibody or cell-mediated immunity.

IMPACTIONS: Bowel pockets formed by gas pressure or faeces impacted onto the colon wall retaining putrefactive matter which is not eliminated in daily bowel movements.

IN VITRO: A Latin term for studies done in test tubes.

INFLAMMATION: The reaction of body tissue to injury or infection characterized by heat, redness, swelling and pain.

INTERFERON: A protein formed by the cells of the immune system in the presence of a virus, etc. It prevents viral reproduction, and is capable of protecting non-infected cells from viral infection. Several kinds of interferon exist including alpha, beta, and gamma.

IRIS: The coloured muscular diaphragm in the eye that surrounds and controls the size of the pupil, and reflects and affects the tissues throughout the body.

KREBS CYCLE: Famous metabolic cycle discovered by Hans Krebs of England, a Nobel prize winner. This refers to the metabolic pathway in which carbohydrates are broken down into energy.

LACTASE: An enzyme that aids the body in converting lactose to glucose and galactose. It is also necessary for digestion of milk and milk products.

LACUNA(E): A 'hole' seen in the iris fibres which may appear in a variety of shapes and sizes and indicate inherent weakness in the tissue.

LECITHIN: A mixture of phospholipids that is composed of fatty acids, glycerol, phosphorus, and choline or inositol. Lecithin can be manufactured in the body. All living cell membranes are largely composed of lecithin.

LIPID: Fat or fatty substance.

LIPOPROTEIN: Fatty substances (fats, oils, cholesterol, carotene, vitamin E) carried in an envelope made of protein and phospholipid (lecithin-like) materials. Specifically, it refers to transport vehicles for fats and cholesterol in our blood and lymph fluids. Lipoproteins carry lipids between our intestine, liver, and body cells.

LONG-CHAIN FATTY ACID: A fatty acid containing more than 14 carbon atoms in its chain.

LOW-DENSITY LIPOPROTEINS (LDL): Vehicles that transport fats and cholesterol via the bloodstream to the cells. An excess of these vehicles is said by medical dogma to be associated with cardiovascular disease; hence it is also called the 'bad' cholesterol. When measured separately from apo(a), LDL is only a mild risk factor. See also: lipoprotein(a).

LYMPH: A clear fluid that flows through lymph vessels and is collected from the tissues throughout the body. Its function is to nourish tissue cells and return waste matter to the bloodstream. The lymph system eventually connects with and adds to venous circulation.

LYMPH GLANDS: Located in the lymph vessels of the body, these glands trap foreign material and produce lymphocytes. These glands act as filters in the lymph system, and contain and form lymphocytes and permit lymphatic cells to destroy certain foreign agents.

LYMPHATIC ROSARY: A string of small puffy clouds in the lymphatic zone of the iris that range in colour from white to yellow to brown and indicate congestion of the lymphatic system and an excess of mucus.

LYMPHOCYTE: A type of white blood cell without certain granules; it numbers from 25 to 30 percent of total white cells in normal individuals found in lymph, blood, and other specialized tissue such as bone marrow and tonsils. B- and T-lymphocytes are crucial components of the immune system. The B-lymphocytes are primarily responsible for antibody production. The T-lymphocytes are involved in the direct attack against invading organisms. The helper T-lymphocytes, a subtype, is the main cell infected and destroyed by the AIDS virus.

MACROPHAGE: A cell able to engulf foreign particulate substances.

MEDIUM-CHAIN TRIGLYCERIDES (MCT): Artificial fat molecules made from a fraction of tropical oils that contain mostly 8- and 10-carbon saturated fatty acids as well as some 6- and 12-carbon chains.

METABOLIC PATHWAY: The way in which energy is taken from protein, fat or carbohydrate. There are thousands of metabolic pathways in the body. The main ones are the carbohydrate (Krebs) and fatty acid cycles. Protein mainly uses the carbohydrate pathway.

METABOLISM: The chemical processes of living cells in which energy is produced in order to replace and repair tissues and maintain a healthy body. Responsible for the production of energy, biosynthesis of important substances, and degradation of various compounds.

METABOLITE: A product or part of a metabolic pathway.

MICROBE: A micro-organism (e.g. bacterium, fungus, virus, protozoan).

MICRONUTRIENT: A nutrient needed by the body in extremely small quantities (e.g. we need calcium in large quantities, and it is called a macronutrient).

MILLILITRES (mL): Thousandths of a litre; same as cubic centimetre.

MILLIMOLES PER LITRE (mmol/L): New measure used by doctors for determining serum cholesterol. Metric Système International (SI).

MOLECULE: A minute mass of matter; smallest quantity into which a substance can be divided and retain its characteristic properties.

MUCOUS MEMBRANES: The membranes, such as in the mouth, nose, anus, and vagina, that line the cavities and canals of the body which communicate with the air.

MUTAGEN: An agent able to induce cell mutation, a step along the cancer process.

MYCOPLASMA: Type of bacteria which possesses no true cell wall.

NATURAL KILLER CELLS: NK cells recognize and kill invaders without any known antigenic stimulation and without any antibody to the invaders.

NATUROPATHY: System of remedial treatment based upon the vital healing force within nature and within mankind, which seeks to support and strengthen that force by natural means.

NERVE RINGS: Also referred to as cramp rings and tension rings seen as

circular contractions of iris fibres and indicating the accumulation of physiological and emotional stress and tension.

NEUROTRANSMITTER: These are often made up of amino acids or peptides
and refer to chemical languages by which cells (neurons) of the brain
communicate with each other. As we speak different languages, so do cells
speak to each other in different languages.

OIL: A liquid fat. The shorter the fatty acid chains or the more omega 3 or
omega 6 double bonds present in them, the more liquid the oil.

OLEIC: An 18-carbon mono-unsaturated fatty acid found in olive, peanut,
canola, pecan, macadamia, and other oils.

OMEGA 3: Fatty acids essential to human health, our bodies make prostaglandins, which prevent the negative effects of series 2 prostaglandins by
preventing their production.

OMEGA 6: A related fatty acid essential for human health, the body makes
series 1 and series 2 prostaglandins. Excess of the latter can cause inflammation, water retention, increased blood pressure, sticky platelets and
decreased immune response.

OMEGA 6:3 BALANCE: The balance of omega 6 to omega 3 fatty acids that
leads to optimum health. Three omega 6 to each omega 3 might be considered a good balance, and is provided by hemp seed oil.

OPEN LACUNAE: Lacunae beginning toward ANW and opening outwards. It
indicates that whilst the organ is weak, it is still receiving adequate nutrients and is able to eliminate metabolic wastes.

ORTHOMOLECULAR: Of the right molecules. In nutrition, it is the maintenance of health and the treatment of disease by varying the concentrations
of substances normally present in the body (vitamins, minerals, fatty acids,
amino acids, enzymes, hormones).

OXIDATION: A chemical reaction that occurs when oxygen is added, resulting
in a chemical transformation.

OXIDIZE: The addition of oxygen, subtraction of hydrogen, or addition of
electrons to a substance, often accompanied by a release of energy.

PARASITE: An organism that lives off another organism.

PARTIALLY HYDROGENATED: An oil in which some but not all double
bonds have been destroyed by adding hydrogen to the fatty acid molecules
under pressure and high temperature in the presence of a nickel-aluminium
catalyst. A semi-solid plastic fat results. Many chemical changes take place
in the fatty acid molecules during this process.

PEPTIDE: A link between two amino acids. Peptide refers to two or more
amino acids.

PEROXIDE VALUE (PV): A measure of rancidity in oils.

PEROXIDES: Free radicals that are by-products formed in our bodies when
molecules of fat react with oxygen.

PHAGOCYTES: Cells that kill, remove, and dispose of invading microbes.

PHENYLALANINE (PHe): An essential amino acid.

PHOSPHOLIPID: A substance consisting primarily of fatty acids and phosphorus, such as lecithin, occurring in all membranes.

PLATELET: Small, colourless disks in circulating blood, which aid in blood
clotting. Platelets become more sticky (form clots easier) when we consume
hard or hydrogenated fats, and less sticky (form clots less readily) when we
consume essential fatty acids.

POLYCHLORINATED BIPHENYL (PCB): Organic (aromatic) molecules that have been reacted with chlorine. Such molecules are extremely toxic, and also cause cancer.

POLYETHYLENE (PE): A type of plastic that is acceptable packaging material for foods and oils. Many plastics are toxic and therefore should not be used to package foods.

POLYUNSATURATED FATTY ACID (PUFA): A fatty acid that contains more than one double bond between carbon atoms in its chain. The term includes both natural, health-enhancing as well as unnatural, health-destroying kinds.

PRECURSOR: Parent substance; a substance out of which another substance is made by chemical modification.

PREMENSTRUAL SYNDROME (PMS): A nutrition-related degenerative condition affecting women before the onset of the monthly period. Water retention, bloating, mood swings, and behavioural difficulties are often involved.

PRESERVATIVE: Any of a large number of possible compounds that slow down chemical deterioration.

PROSTAGLANDIN (PG): A fatty acid partially oxidized in a very specific and controlled way by enzymes made in the body for just this purpose. Prostaglandins have hormone-like functions in the regulation of cell activity. Over 30 different prostaglandins are known.

PROTEIN: Protein is one of the building blocks of the body. A group of complex molecules with specific and precise structural and chemical functions. They are made by linking together amino acids in a specific linear sequence and then folding these chains in particular 3-dimensional ways.

PUPIL: The dark circular aperture at the centre of the iris through which light enters the inner eye.

RADII SOLARIS: Spikes emanating from the intestinal zone (caused by impactions) and the ANW indicating a possible reflex disturbance to the area of the body to which the spike is pointing.

RETINA: The light-sensitive membrane forming the inner lining of the posterior wall of the eyeball composed largely of specialized terminal expansions of the optic nerve.

RIBONUCLEIC ACID (RNA): Messages translated from genetic material (DNA), that are used by our cells to synthesize proteins.

SATURATED FATTY ACID (SaFa): A fatty acid with no double bonds in the carbon chain, and with every possible position on the carbon atoms taken up by hydrogen atoms.

SCLERA: The white of the eye surrounding the iris.

SCURF RIM: A darkening in the skin zone of the iris due to the retention of wastes, suppression and inactivity of the skin.

SEROTONIN: A major neurotransmitter in the brain made from tryptophan, present in nerve tissue. Considered essential for relaxation, sleep, and concentration.

SHORT-CHAIN FATTY ACIDS: A fatty acid with 6 or less carbon atoms in its chain.

SIMPLE CARBOHYDRATES: A simple sugar. Glucose, fructose and lactose are examples, as well as sucrose (table sugar). Simple carbohydrates are absorbed into the bloodstream rapidly.

SPORES: Reproductive cells of certain lower organisms, such as the tetanus germ, covered by a thick shell, which survives great heat and cold. Difficult to destroy.

STARCH: Glucose molecules hooked together into branching chains by plant cells. Digested and absorbed slowly, starches supply energy at the rate at which the body uses it.

STEARIC ACID: An 18-carbon saturated fatty acid abundant in hard fats.

STOMACH HALO: A circular white/silver halo in the stomach zone around the pupil.

SUPEROXIDE DISMUTASE (SOD): An enzyme made in our body that neutralizes free radicals that could otherwise cause damage to cells.

SYSTEMIC INFECTION: Condition wherein bacteria or other organisms invade the blood and/or internal organs.

T AND B CELLS: White cells, derived from the thymus gland and bone marrow, respectively.

T-CELL: A type of lymphocyte crucial to the immune system and involved in the direct attack upon invading organisms.

T-HELPER CELLS: White cells that attack an invading organism.

T-HELPER TO T-SUPPRESSOR RATIO: The ratio of T-helper to T-suppressor cells, normally about 1.8:1 in healthy individuals.

T-SUPPRESSOR CELLS: White cells that stop the action of T-helper cells once the invaders have been destroyed. When T-suppressor cells increase disproportionately in number, they may destroy our ability to fight infection, hence destroying our immune system.

THRUSH: A fungal infection from Candida albicans. Occurs most often in infants, immunocompromised patients, and AIDS victims. Characterized by small whitish spots on the tongue and inside of the cheeks.

TOPHI (tophus): Discolourations in the iris resembling flakes, clouds or spots that range from white to yellow in colour and indicate congestion.

TOXICITY: A poisonous reaction in the body that impairs bodily functions and/or damages cells. Caused from ingesting an amount of a substance that is higher than one's level of tolerance.

TOXINS: Accumulation of pollutants, body wastes, minerals, drugs and chemicals which collect in the blood and lymph and put a stress on all the eliminative channels of the body.

TRANSVERSALS: White or vascularized acute signs which run across the normal fibre direction, indicating adhesions, and acute to chronic irritability. (see IRIS)

TRANVERSE COLON: The section of the colon which goes across the upper abdomen between the liver on the right-hand side and the spleen on the left.

TRIGLYCERIDE: A compound consisting of glycerol and a fatty acid. Triglycerides are fat storage molecules and are the major lipid component of the diet.

VIRUS: Any of a vast group of minute structures composed of a protein coat and a core of DNA and/or RNA that reproduces in the cells of the infected host. Capable of infecting all animals and plants, causing devastating disease in immunocompromised individuals. Viruses are not affected by antibiotics, and are totally dependent on the cells of the infected host for the ability to reproduce.

VITAMIN: Approximately fifteen essential nutrients that the body cannot manufacture and that need to be supplied for life and health.

YEAST: Yeast is a single-cell organism that may cause infection in the mouth, vagina, gastro-intestinal tract, and any or all bodily parts. Common yeast infections include Candidiasis and thrush.

Notes

Chapter 2. Food

1. Robbins, John, *Diet for a New America* (1987)
2. Pearson, D., and Shaw, S., 'Spices and other Foods', *Life Extension*, Part IV, Chapter 3, p. 383
3. Wigmore, Ann, *The Wheatgrass Book* (Avery Publishing Group, Inc., Wayne, New Jersey, 1985)
4. Blauer, Stephen, *Rejuvenation (Dr Harvey Lisle 'Letter to Ann Wigmore')* (Green Grown Publications, USA, 1980 p. 105)

Chapter 3. Digestion and Elimination

5. Mindell, Earl, *Earl Mindell's Vitamin Bible* (Raveson, Wade Publishers, Inc., New York, 1979)
6. Gray, Henry F.R.S., *Gray's Anatomy, Descriptive and Surgical* (Crown Publishers, Inc., 1977 pp. 554–6).

Chapter 4. Colon Maintenance

7. De Schepper, Luc, M.D., *Peak Immunity* (Dr Luc De Schepper, Santa Monica, California, 1989 p. 103)

Chapter 5. Iridology

8. Jensen, Bernard, Dr, *The Science and Practice of Iridology* (B. Jensen, 1952)
9. Jackson, Adam, J. *Alternative Health Iridology* (Macdonald & Co London)
10. Kriege, T., *Fundamental Basis of Iris Diagnosis* (L.N. Fowler & Co. Ltd., 1985)

Chapter 6. Amino Acids

11. Brauerman, Eric R., *The Healing Nutrients Within: Facts, Findings and New Research on Amino Acids* (Keats Publishing, Inc., 1987)
12. Erdmann, Robert, *The Amino Revolution* (Robert Ergmann with Merrion Jones, Fireside, 1987)
13. Brauerman, Eric R., *The Healing Nutrients Within: Facts, Findings and New Research on Amino Acids* (Keats Publishing, Inc., 1987)

Chapter 8. Cell Salts

14. Boerick and Dewey, *The Twelve Tissue Remedies of Schussler* (B. Jain Publishers Put. Ltd, Delhi, Reprint Edition 1993)

Chapter 9. Homeopathy

15. Boericke, William, MD, *Homeopathic Materia Medica* (Motibal Banarsidass Publishers, Delhi, 1993)

16. Schepper, Luc de, M.D., Ph.D, *Human Condition Critical* (Full of Life Publishing, New Mexico, USA 1993 p. 122)

Chapter 10. Electrolytes

17. Prof Muller, *Elements of Physiology*

18. Smith, Lendon H., *Feed your Body Right* (M. Evans and Company, Inc., New York, 1994 p. 148)

Chapter 11. Free Radicals

19. *Clinical Pearls* 1992 p. 457

20. Pearson, Dirk and Shaw, Sandy, *The Life Extension Companion* (Warner Books, Inc. NY, 1984 p. 103

21. *Clinical Pearls* 1993 p. 273

22. Weiner, Michael A. Ph.D., *Maximum Immunity* (Pocket books, London, 1986)

23. Halliwell, Barry, M.D. et al., 'Free Radicals, Antioxidants and Human Disease: Where are we now?' *Journal of Laboratory and Clinical Medicine*, 119 (1992) pp. 598-620

24. Pearson, Dirk and Shaw, Sandy, *Life Extension* (Warner Books, Inc., New York, 1982 p. 103)

25. Balch, Jr., James and Balch, Phyllis A., *Prescription for Nutritional Healing* (Avery Publishing Group, Inc. 1990 p. 96)

26. McGrady, Sr. Pat, *The Persecuted Drug, The Story of DMSO* (Charter Books, New York, 1973)

27. Emerit, Ingrid, *Free Radicals and Aging of the Skin* (Birkhauser Verlag, Basel, Switzerland, 1992 pp. 338-340)

28. Pearson, Dirk and Shaw, Sandy, *The Life Extension Companion* (Warner Books, Inc. NY, 1984 p. 484)

29. Pearson, Dirk and Shaw, Sandy, *The Life Extension Companion* (Warner Books, Inc. NY, 1984 p. 473)

30. Edes, Thomas E., M.D., 'Beta Carotene and Vitamin A: Casting Separate Shadows?', *The Nutrition Report*, 10 (1992) pp. 9–16

31. Thurnham, David I., 'Carotenoids: Function and Fallacies', *Proceedings of the Nutritional Society*, 53 (1994) pp. 77–87

32. *Clinical Pearls* 1992 p. 458 KE Cartenoids Glutathione

33. *Clinical Pearls* 1992 p. 279 Glutathione Metabolism

34. *Clinical Pearls* 1992 p. 305 Methionine feeding

35. Pearson, Dirk and Shaw, Sandy, *The Life Extension Companion* (Warner Books, Inc. NY, 1984 p. 474) and *Clinical Pearls* 1992 p. 282, Effect of B6

36. Pearson, Dirk and Shaw, Sandy, *The Life Extension Companion* (Warner Books, Inc. NY, 1984 p. 481)

37. Pearson, Dirk and Shaw, Sandy, *The Life Extension Companion* (Warner Books, Inc. NY, 1984 p. 470)

38. Pearson, Dirk and Shaw, Sandy, *The Life Extension Companion* (Warner Books, Inc. NY, 1984 p. 471)

39. *The Miracle Nutrient CoQ[10]* – Emile Bliznakor, MD

40. Baur, A. et al. 'Alpha-Lipoic acid is an effective inhibitor of Human Immunodeficiency Virus (HIV-1) replication'. *Klin Wochenscher* 69 1991 pp. 722–4.

Wickramasinghe, S.N. and Hasan, R., 'In Vitro Effects of Vitamin C, Thioctic Acid and Dihydrolipoic Acid on the Cytotoxicity of Post-Ethanol Serum'. *Biochemical Pharmacology* (1992) pp. 407–11.

Chapter 12. Blood Chemistry

41. Gomella, Leonard G., *Clinicians Pocket Reference* (Prentice Hall International (UK) Limited, London, Seventh Edition, 1993)

42. Golper, Thomas A., and Suhail A., 'L-Carnitine' *Clinical Pearls* (1992) p. 406

43. Beisel, et al, 1981

44. Rosenbaum, 1984

45. *Healing Nutrients Within*, p. 381

46. Pearson, Dirk and Shaw, Sandy, *The Life Extension Companion* (Warner Books, Inc. NY, 1984 p. 304)

47. De Schepper, Luc M.D., PhD. *Human Condition Critical* (Full of Life Publishing, New Mexico, USA, 1993)

48. Clark, Hulda, Regehr, PhD., N.D. *The cure for all Cancers* (Pro Motion Publishing, Calif., USA, 1993)

Chapter 13. Parasites

49. *Clinical Pearls*, research article p. 377 'Parasites by State Diagnostic Laboratories'

50. Stauric, B. and Matula. T.T., 'Flavanoids in Foods: Their significance for Nutrition and Health', *Lipid Soluable Antioxidants, Biochemistry and Clinical Applications.* (Bureau of Chemical Safety, Ottowa, Ontario 1992 pp. 274-94)

51. Baskerville, A., Hambleton, P., Benbough, J.E., 'Pathological features of Glutaminase Toxicity' *Br J Exp Pathol* (1980) pp. 132-8

52. Neursholme, E.A., Crabtree, B., Ardavie, M.S.M., England. 'Glutamine Metabolism in Lymphocytes: Its Biochemical, Physiological and Clinical importance'

53. Hurley, Dan, 'Beta-Carotene may Detoxify Carcinogens', *Medical Tribune*, August 20, 1992 p. 24

54. Nagabhushan, M., Ph.D 'Curcumin as an Inhibitor of Cancer', and Bhide, S.V., *Journal of the American College of Nutrition* 11 (1992) pp. 192-8

55. Bast, A. and Henen, G., 'Interplay between lipoic acid and glutathione in protection against microsomal lipid peroxidation'. *Bioch et Biophys*, Acta 963 (1988) pp. 558-62

56. 'Decreased resistance to antibiotics and plasmid loss in plasmid-carrying strains of Staphlococcus aureus treated with ascorbic acid'. *Mutation Research* 264 (1991) pp. 119-25

57. Weaver, Leon D. VMD, *Antibiotic Residues in Milk and Meat: Perception and Realities.* University of California, Davis, 1992 pp. 1222-8

58. Ingram, Cass, D.O., *A Disaster Survival Guide* (Literary Visions Publishing, Inc., 1992)

59. Bradford, Robert and Rodriguez, Rodrigo, M.D., of the American Biologics – Mexico S.A. Research Hospital, Tijuana, B.C., Mexico

60. Hill, R., 1977 *Propolis – The natural antibiotic* (Thorsons Publishers Limited, England)

61. Belanche, P., 'Treatment of skin infections with essential oil of Melaluca alternifolia' *Pytotherapie* 15 (1985) pp. 15-17

Chapter 14. HIV

62. Gallo C., *Virus Hunting, Aids, Cancer and the Human Retrovirus: A Story of Human Discovery* (A New Republic Book, Basic Books, 1991)

Conclusion

63. Hippeli, Sussanne and Elstner, Erich, *Oxygen Radicals and Air Pollution* (1991 Chapter 1 pp. 3-55)

64. Pearson, Dirk and Shaw, Sandy, *The Life Extension Companion* (Warner Books, Inc. NY, 1984, p. 119)

65. Sackler Arthur M., *Medical Tribune*, 9/18/1985, p. 46

Acknowledgements

I began writing this book three years ago. My intention was to pass on the fruits of my research and the experience of my patients over the years. Knowledge is useless unless it is shared.

Many people have encouraged me in this process. My mother taught me courage and strength. My sister Delveen worked untiringly preparing the typescript. Martin Taylor edited the typescript meticulously for press. Brian Sullivan encouraged me throughout with his great enthusiasm. Diana for helping get it published.

Finally I thank James Cordell for his unconditional support and friendship.

Note

The procedures and suggestions in this book are not intended as a substitute for the medical advice of a health professional. All matters regarding your health that require diagnosis or medical attention should be dealt with under medical supervision. The author and publishers disclaim any liability arising directly or indirectly from the use of this book.

For further information relating to this book please write to:

Health Spectrum
149 Columbia Drive
Rancho Mirage, CA 92270